Video Displays, Work, and Vision

Panel on Impact of Video Viewing
on Vision of Workers

Committee on Vision

Commission on Behavioral and
Social Sciences and Education

National Research Council

NATIONAL ACADEMY PRESS
Washington, D.C.   1983

This work relates to the Department of the Navy Contract N00014-81-C-0422 issued by the Office of Naval Research under Contract Authority NR 201-517. However, the content does not necessarily reflect the position or the policy of the Department of the Navy or the government, and no official endorsement should be inferred.

The United States government has at least a royalty-free, nonexclusive, and irrevocable license throughout the world for government purposes to publish, translate, reproduce, deliver, perform, dispose of, and to authorize others so to do, all or any portion of this work.

Library of Congress Catalog Card Number 83-61880
International Standard Book Number 0-309-03388-8

NATIONAL ACADEMY PRESS
2101 Constitution Avenue, NW
Washington, DC 20418

Panel on Impact of Video Viewing on Vision of Workers

EDWARD J. RINALDUCCI (*Chair*), School of Psychology, Georgia Institute of Technology
JANET BERTINUSON, Alberta Federation of Labour
ROBERT D. CAPLAN, Institute for Social Research, University of Michigan
ROBERT M. GUION, Department of Psychology, Bowling Green State University
VINCENT M. KING, College of Optometry, Ferris State College
DAVID H. SLINEY, Laser Branch, U.S. Army Environmental Hygiene Agency
STANLEY W. SMITH, Institute for Research in Vision, Ohio State University
HARRY L. SNYDER, Department of Industrial Engineering and Operations Research, Virginia Polytechnic Institute and State University
ALFRED SOMMER, International Center for Epidemiologic and Preventive Ophthalmology, Wilmer Ophthalmological Institute, Johns Hopkins University
LAWRENCE W. STARK, Neurology Unit, University of California, Berkeley
H. LEE TASK, Air Force Aerospace Medical Research Laboratory, Wright-Patterson Air Force Base
HUGH R. TAYLOR, International Center for Epidemiologic and Preventive Ophthalmology, Wilmer Ophthalmological Institute, Johns Hopkins University

Staff

KEY DISMUKES, Study Director
BARBARA S. BROWN, Staff Associate
LLYN M. ELLISON, Administrative Secretary
GRAY JACOBIK, Secretary

Committee on Vision

Preface

In the spring of 1981 the National Institute for Occupational Safety and Health (NIOSH) requested the National Academy of Sciences to undertake a critical review of existing studies of visual issues encountered in occupational video viewing, analyze methodological problems, and suggest lines of research to resolve remaining questions. In response to this request, the National Research Council's Committee on Vision established the Panel on Impact of Video Viewing on Vision of Workers, which has prepared this report.

The National Research Council appointed panel members with expertise in the diverse scientific and technical areas relevant to occupational video viewing, in particular, ophthalmology, optometry, oculomotor function, physiological optics, epidemiology, occupational health, radiation biophysics, display technology, illuminating engineering, human factors, and industrial and organizational psychology. The areas of expertise of individual panel members are described in Appendix D.

This report focuses on the six issues that NIOSH asked the panel to address:

1. How well are the visual factors and underlying mechanisms that produce discomfort in video viewing understood?

2. What problems are encountered in attempting to define "eyestrain" and "visual fatigue" and to relate physiological, subjective, ergonomic, and performance measures of these concepts?

3. Is existing knowledge sufficient to establish adequate standards for display characteristics (contrast ratios, luminance levels, regeneration rate, etc.)? Is there an adequate basis for standardizing viewing conditions, such as the portion of operators' time spent viewing video display terminals?

4. To what extent are the problems reported with video terminals due to substandard operating conditions (e.g., excessive glare from overhead

illumination), and to what extent would these problems remain even under ideal viewing conditions?

5. What can be said about the relative roles of visual, ergonomic, and psychosocial factors in visual problems encountered? What can be said about the relation of visual symptoms encountered and more general stress responses (e.g., general fatigue) to other aspects of the worker's job?

6. How do visual problems in video viewing compare with those encountered in comparable tasks, such as prolonged editing or typing of print?

Because many workers and labor union representatives have been concerned that radiation hazards may be associated with the use of video display terminals (VDTs), the panel also decided to consider radiation issues in its work.

In the course of its study the panel reviewed diverse literatures, including reports of field surveys of VDT workers and VDT workplaces, laboratory studies of visual functions in VDT work tasks, news articles, and pamphlets prepared by labor unions concerned with VDT issues. The panel also drew upon the substantial technical literatures on visual function, image quality, lighting design, ergonomic design, and industrial and organizational psychology that are highly germane but often neglected in discussions of VDT issues.

To further its discussions of technical issues and to promote the exchange of information among scientists and representatives of labor, industry, and federal agencies, the panel held a public symposium on video display terminals and vision of workers on August 20-21, 1981, in Washington, D.C. (summarized by Brown et al., 1982). Investigators from around the world were invited to present their research on VDTs and to review field surveys of VDT workers. Discussion panels included scientists, who analyzed technical aspects of VDT studies, and labor representatives, who described the concerns of workers. The panel has drawn on the symposium presentations and discussions in analyzing the issues discussed in this report.

The panel recognized early in its deliberations that visual issues in VDT work must be considered within the larger context of the working environment, including the quality of VDT workstation equipment, job design, and workers' concerns and needs for information. This larger context was discussed extensively at the panel's meetings and is considered explicitly in this report.

Early drafts of material were prepared for the panel's review and discussion by panel members, consultants, and staff. The panel's analyses of survey methodology and of psychosocial issues were prepared by Robert Caplan and Robert Guion. Janet Bertinuson provided guidance on characteristics of various types of working situations in which VDTs are used and on the concerns of the labor community. David Sliney reviewed surveys of radiation emissions, and Alfred Sommer and Hugh R. Taylor analyzed issues involving epidemiology and cataracts. Vincent King, Edward Rinalducci, Stanley Smith, Harry Snyder, and Lee Task prepared material on lighting and reflections and display technology. Panel consultants Martin Helander and K. H. E. Kroemer drafted material on human factors for the panel's discussion. Key Dismukes prepared material on visual tasks and symptoms in VDT work, drawing in part upon ideas and material contributed by NRC fellow Raymond Briggs, Committee on Vision member Julian Hochberg, and consultant John Merritt. Lawrence Stark reviewed the literature on oculomotor factors affecting visual performance. Phyllis Johnston, at the University of California, Berkeley, assisted in reviewing the literature on oculomotor functions. Harry Snyder and Martin Helander provided information on current guidelines and standards for VDT use. Consultant R. Van Harrison provided a review and critique of the NIOSH *Baltimore Sun* study, which appears as Appendix B. Barbara S. Brown and Key Dismukes prepared the summary chapter.

All members of the panel were asked to critically review drafts of the report chapters, all of which were then discussed at panel meetings. The chapters were then revised accordingly, and at its final meeting in February 1982 the panel summarized its conclusions. Thus the study and the report are a collaborative effort of all members of the panel and the staff.

The panel also benefited from thoughtful reviews of early drafts of this report by members of the Committee on Vision and the Commission on Behavioral and Social Sciences and Education and other experts, whose comments the panel drew upon in preparing the final version. Julian Hochberg provided valuable insights on conceptual issues throughout the course of the study and contributed to the development of the entire report; Derek Fender made helpful comments and suggestions on the entire report and contributed to the panel's discussion of several key issues; and several other members of the committee, in particular Anthony Adams, Eliot L. Berson, Dorothea Jameson, and Luis Proenza, provided helpful comments and suggestions. The committee was assisted in its review by comments solicited from David Cogan, at the National Eye Institute; Arthur Jampolsky, at the Smith-Kettlewell Institute of Visual Sciences; and Donald Pitts, at the University of Houston.

Barbara S. Brown played a substantial and invaluable role, collaborating with us to coordinate and manage the study. In addition, she organized and edited drafts of technical material, wrote supplementary material, and helped integrate the discussion of issues in the report. She also helped organize the panel's symposium and meetings.

Llyn M. Ellison provided expert administrative and secretarial assistance throughout the study. She took care of many administrative details, helped arrange meetings, and was centrally involved in preparing the manuscript for production. In the process of efficiently and expertly producing manuscript drafts on a VDT, she gained firsthand experience in some of the concerns of VDT workers. Gray Jacobik assisted with secretarial tasks and word processing. We are grateful for their skillful assistance. Eugenia Grohman, on the staff of the Commission on Behavioral and Social Sciences and Education, gave helpful advice on organizing the material in the report and expertly edited the final version.

EDWARD J. RINALDUCCI, *Chair*

KEY DISMUKES, *Study Director*
Panel on Video Viewing

Contents

Executive Summary

The issues we were requested to address in this study are presented in the preface. Our findings and conclusions respond both to these issues and to related issues and concerns that we considered in our work.

Although much has been written in the last several years about the problems and concerns of people who work with video display terminals (VDTs), the literature has been based predominantly on a small number of studies, many of which have substantial short-comings in methodology that severely limit the conclusions that can appropriately be drawn from them. In addition to reviewing that literature, we have drawn upon substantial technical literatures on visual function, image quality, lighting design, ergonomic design, and industrial and organizational psychology. To a large extent our conclusions are based on these more extensive and better validated literatures.

1. Surveys of workers who use VDTs indicate that complaints and symptoms of job-related ocular discomfort, musculoskeletal discomfort, and stress are common. Surveys that have included comparison groups of non-VDT workers suggest that the frequency of such complaints is greater among workers who use VDTs than among those who do not. Most surveys, however, have been poorly designed, and the inferences that may reasonably be drawn from them are suggestive rather than conclusive. Surveys have not established whether complaints and reported symptoms are related to VDT characteristics, other aspects of the workplace and job situation, or some combination of these factors. Most studies have not adequately considered the heterogeneity of VDT job situations. Evidence suggests that job design and task require-ments can produce job-related physical symptoms and stress. Thus it is possible that differences in reported symptoms between VDT workers and non-VDT workers might be more directly related to characteristics of the work situation--i.e., the way in which

1

VDTs are used--than to characteristics inherent in VDTs. Given the lack of adequate controls in survey studies, the relative influence of equipment characteristics and job characteristics remains an open question.

2. The comfort, performance, levels of stress, and job satisfaction of workers who regularly use VDTs have in many cases been adversely affected by failure to apply to jobs and equipment well-established principles of good design and practice. A considerable literature exists on the effects of image display characteristics on legibility and user performance, and well-designed, high-quality VDTs are available commercially. In many instances, however, VDTs have been designed without attention to existing scientific data on image quality, and many VDTs on the market do not provide the legibility of high-quality printed material. In addition, in many instances VDTs have been introduced into workplaces with little attention to principles of human factors, illuminating engineering, and industrial and organizational psychology. We strongly recommend that manu-facturers and users of VDT equipment draw upon available scientific data in designing and selecting VDT equipment and in designing VDT-related work.

3. The terms visual fatigue and eyestrain are frequently used in ill-defined and differing ways. These terms do not correspond to known physiological or clinical conditions. We suggest instead that researchers and others use terms that specifically describe the phenomena discussed, such as ocular discomfort, changes in visual performance, and changes in oculomotor functions.

4. The symptoms of ocular discomfort and difficulty with vision reported by some workers who use VDTs appear to be similar to symptoms reported by people performing other near-visual tasks. Temporary changes in measures of visual function reported to occur following VDT work appear to be similar to those observed after performance of near-visual tasks in non-VDT jobs. Most features of VDT work tasks that may contribute to discomfort or visual difficulty are also found in various jobs not involving VDTs; however, poorly designed VDTs, workstations, and work tasks, often produce a particularly problematic concatenation of adverse features.

5. It is not known whether ocular discomfort and reported changes in measures of visual function are related. In general, the physiological and psychological mechanisms underlying ocular discomfort are poorly understood. However, there is no scien-tifically valid evidence that ocular discomfort or temporary

changes in visual functions are associated with damage to the visual system.

6. A number of competent studies have found that the levels of radiation emitted by VDTs are far below current U.S. occupational radiation exposure standards and are generally much lower than the ambient radiation emitted by natural and human-made sources to which people are continuously exposed. We have not attempted to evaluate the adequacy of existing standards, but our review of the scientific literature on biological effects of radiation indicates that the levels of radiation emitted by VDTs under conditions of normal operation and under conditions of malfunction or aging of the VDT are highly unlikely to be hazardous. These considerations suggest that routine radiation surveys of VDTs in the workplace are not warranted. However, radiation testing of new VDT models should be continued to ensure that product safety standards are met.

7. We find no scientifically valid evidence that occupational use of VDTs is associated with increased risk of ocular diseases or abnormalities, including cataracts. Existing knowledge makes such an association seem quite unlikely. Only if competent pilot studies were to indicate such an association would large-scale epidemiological studies of cataracts among VDT workers be warranted.

8. We find no scientifically valid evidence that the use of VDTs per se causes harm, in the sense of anatomical or physiological damage, to the visual system. There is nothing in the literature on the effects of working with VDTs, or in the broader realm of existing scientific and clinical knowledge, that suggests that such a causal relationship is likely.

9. It is difficult for manufacturers, purchasers, and users to make meaningful comparisons between VDT products because techniques for measuring image characteristics and evaluating quality have not been standardized and applied in commerce. We recommend that efforts be made to standardize measurement techniques. Characteristic measures of products should be made routinely available to purchasers and users.

10. Existing data do not provide a sufficient basis for establishing mandatory standards for display, lighting, and workstation parameters or for task designs and work schedules in VDT-related work. Research is needed to provide adequate data that can be used as a basis for decisions regarding standards. In the meantime, application of well-established principles of good design and

practice can be expected to reduce the incidence of complaints of work-related physical symptoms and stress and to enhance the comfort and performance of workers.

11. Carefully designed research on the effects of VDT characteristics on visual performance and comfort would be useful, especially in view of the projected increase in the number of workers who will be using such equipment in the future. Research on psychosocial parameters that affect all jobs, such as workload, task complexity, and social support, would seem to offer more potential benefit than research on psychosocial variables specific to VDT work. We emphasize, however, that application of existing knowledge in designing and using VDTs should be given high priority.

1
Summary of Findings

INTRODUCTION

Background

Video display terminals (VDTs)[1] are used in a broad range of
occupations (e.g., clerical work, printing, computer work, air
traffic control), and their use in offices is growing rapidly. The
number of VDT operators in the United States was estimated to be
approximately 7 million in 1980, with 5-10 million VDTs in use
(Center for Disease Control, 1980).

Workers and union representatives around the world have
expressed concern that harmful effects may result from working
with VDTs (see, e.g., Bergman, 1980; New York Committee for
Occupational Safety and Health, 1980; Working Women, National
Association of Office Workers, 1980; DeMatteo et al., 1981;
Canadian Labour Congress, 1982). Much of this concern has
involved visual functions, human factors,[2] radiation, and

---

[1]VDTs are devices for visually displaying (with symbols, graphics,
or both) information that is stored and processed electronically.
Keyboards are commonly used to control the processing and
display of information. Most VDTs now commercially available
use cathode-ray tubes (CRTs) and are similar to television
receivers in their display characteristics; however, VDTs that use
solid-state display devices instead of CRTs are increasingly
coming into use.

[2]Human factors are characteristics of people—for example, size,
shape, ability to see and hear, strength, and mental capacities--
that should be considered in the design of equipment and sociotechnical systems. The effects of design variables on human
performance are studied in the field of human factors in order to
develop and apply principles to improve the effectiveness,

psychosocial aspects of VDT-related work. A number of surveys of VDT operators have reported a high incidence of complaints of visual and musculoskeletal discomfort. In several studies in which various visual functions have been measured, they have been reported to be temporarily altered following work at VDTs. Many workers and labor representatives have expressed concern that VDTs may emit harmful levels of radiation that may cause cataracts and other adverse health effects (Working Women, National Association of Office Workers, 1980; DeMatteo et al., 1981; Canadian Labour Congress, 1982). There have been anecdotal reports that clusters of VDT operators have had spontaneous abortions and miscarriages and have given birth to children with birth defects (Microwave News, 1981). Reports of skin rashes among VDT operators have recently appeared (W. C. Olsen, 1981; Nilsen, 1982). Some types of clerical jobs in which VDTs are used have been characterized by some labor represen- tatives as being more stressful than clerical jobs performed using traditional technologies (Working Women, National Association of Office Workers, 1980; Canadian Labour Congress, 1982).

Focus of the Study

This report primarily concerns issues involving vision and the visual system. However, because factors that affect operator comfort and performance cannot be elucidated by analyzing only the optical characteristics of VDTs, relevant human factors and psychosocial issues are also considered. Because much of the concern about the possibility of radiation hazards has been based on misinformation, we analyze the results of surveys in which the levels of radiation have been measured and compare those levels with ambient levels of radiation emitted by human-made and natural sources and with current standards for occupational exposure. We did not reopen the question of what is an acceptable level of radiation exposure, a question that has been extensively studied and was beyond our mandate. We discuss whether there is evidence that ocular diseases or abnormalities, including cata- racts, are associated with VDT-related work (see Chapters 3 and 7). We discuss only briefly the possibility of disorders that do not involve vision (i.e., effects on pregnancy and skin rashes; see

---

efficiency, safety, and comfort of people who use machines. In Europe this field is referred to as ergonomics and somewhat greater emphasis is given to biomechanics and physiological aspects of work than in the United States. The two terms are used interchangeably in this report.

Chapter 3) because there are few published data and because we lack the appropriate expertise.

Organization of the Report

This chapter is intended to provide a nontechnical review of issues and a summary of the panel's findings. The following chapters provide a more extensive analysis of technical issues and literature. Chapter 2 analyzes issues concerning the methodologies encountered in field studies in which VDT workers were asked to respond to questions about visual and other complaints. Shortcomings in the methodologies of these studies make it difficult to draw firm conclusions about the factors underlying visual complaints and symptoms of workers. The first section of Chapter 3 reviews studies of radiation emissions from VDTs and compares the level of emissions with current occupational standards and background radiation from natural and human-made sources. The second section reviews concerns about cataracts and discusses epidemiological issues. Chapter 4 evaluates what is known about the relationship between specific characteristics of display devices and observers' visual performance, subjective responses, and physiological responses. Chapter 5 analyzes the problems VDT workers sometimes experience with improper workstation lighting and reflections, and Chapter 6 examines the ways in which the comfort and performance of workers are affected by constraints on posture and motion imposed by the physical layout of workstations. Chapter 7 explores what is known about the causes of ocular discomfort and difficulties sometimes reported with vision and discusses the limited efforts that have been made to compare visual tasks in jobs that involve VDTs and jobs that do not. Chapter 8 discusses the influence of job design and organizational factors on the well-being of VDT workers. Chapter 9 presents principles of good design and practice that could alleviate problems encountered in VDT work and discusses the feasibility of standards for VDT design. Last, Chapter 10 discusses research needs.

The Literature Base

The literature related to visual effects of VDTs is growing rapidly. The number of articles published per year went from 1 in 1972 to 43 in 1980 (Matula, 1981). This literature, however, has done little to answer the questions that have been raised. Only a dozen or so formal studies of visual complaints or changes in visual function among VDT workers have been published, and most fail to meet major criteria for acceptable scientific research. The remaining literature on visual effects consists mainly of nontechnical reviews of the concerns of workers, technical discussions of standards for VDT and workstation design, and handbooks for workstation design.

In contrast to the literature on visual effects of VDTs, there is a substantial technical literature on the quality of visual displays, the effective design of lighting, and human factors. We are not aware of any formal studies of job design in VDT-related work.

The Nature of VDT Work

This study considers only VDTs used for the display of alpha-numeric information; it does not consider graphic displays (e.g., air traffic control scopes, radar scopes). Nevertheless, the kinds of jobs in which alphanumeric VDTs are used must be at least in the hundreds and include both clerical and professional occupations. These jobs, of course, differ greatly on many dimensions: in the function of the VDT within the job as a whole, in the amount of time the worker spends on tasks in which the VDT is directly involved, in the visual tasks required, etc. It seems likely that the nature and incidence of visual and other problems would vary greatly among diverse VDT jobs; thus, generalizations should be made with caution.

Unfortunately, there has been no formal analysis of task characteristics in various VDT jobs, and there is no ready classification scheme for such jobs. To illustrate the diversity among jobs in which VDTs are used, we can characterize some jobs by a predominant mode of interaction with the VDT (see Table 1.1).

In data entry work, information that is usually noncontextual (numbers, letters, or symbols) is keyed into the computer, often in a repetitive manner according to a set format. In many cases the data have no intrinsic meaning, especially when specialized symbols are used. The work pace in data entry is often quite high--8,000-12,000 keystrokes/h is not unusual (Grandjean, 1980)--and VDT operators may be expected to meet production quotas. Operators may read from printed or handwritten material or use auditory sources. In many cases the task does not require that the operator often look at the video screen. Operators in jobs that primarily involve data entry work usually have little or no control over the structure of their work.

Data acquisition involves calling up information from the computer and reading it from the screen; it is thus more screen-intensive (attention is directed primarily to the screen) than data entry work. Telephone information operators often work predominantly in this mode.

TABLE 1.1 Some Video Display Terminal Task Categories

Task Category	Input Rate (Strokes/Min)	Visual Emphasis	Interruptions	Work Speed Control	Decision Making
Data entry	High	Source document (screen/copy/screen checks)	Very few	Little to none	Little
Data acquisition	Medium	Screen only	Some	Varies	Some
Interactive communication	Medium/intermittent	Screen only (some keyboard)	Lags for processing	Varies	Some
Word processing	High/intermittent	Screen/copy	Few	Some	Varies
Programming	Low/intermittent	Copy/screen	Frequent	Much	Great
CAD/CAM	Low/intermittent	Screen/copy	Frequent	Much	Great

Interactive communication (sometimes called conversational) work involves both data entry and data acquisition. The data may be more complicated than those involved in data entry jobs, and the task is likely to be more screen-intensive. To some degree an operator sustains a dialogue with the computer and has some opportunity for decision making. Airline reservation clerks are an example of workers who seem to work predominantly in this mode.

Word processing involves text entry, text recall, searching text for errors, keying in corrections, and organizing format. The term is often used to refer to secretarial tasks in document preparation, but there are similar operations in such job tasks as layout, formatting, proofreading, and editing. Some of the task elements are source-document-intensive, some are screen-intensive, and word processing jobs usually involve different combinations of these elements at different times. There is wide variation among these jobs in the degree of control an operator may have over the structure and pace of work.

Programming, computer-assisted design (CAD), and computer-assisted manufacturing (CAM) involve some aspect of programming computers using VDTs. Many professional jobs--for example, data analysis, computer programming, scientific research--include such use of VDTs. In these jobs the VDT may be only one of several tools used, and the amount of time a worker spends at a terminal often varies greatly from day to day. A worker's control over the job task is considerable.

Obviously many jobs have elements of more than one of these categories, and some jobs may not fit into any of them.

The comfort, satisfaction, and performance of VDT workers are affected by interacting factors that range from optical to psychosocial (see Figure 1.1). Unfortunately, the existing literature on the effects of VDTs has done little to distinguish the relative contributions of these factors. And VDT jobs have not been systematically analyzed and compared with non-VDT jobs. Furthermore, many jobs have been substantially altered by the introduction of VDTs; and it is difficult to determine from existing data whether reported visual problems and other concerns of workers result from the new technology itself or the way in which it is being introduced.

FIELD STUDIES OF VDT WORKERS AND WORKSTATIONS

Studies of Radiation Emission from VDTs

Video display terminals are designed to emit visible radiation (light), but in the process of producing visible light small amounts of several other types of electromagnetic radiation are also

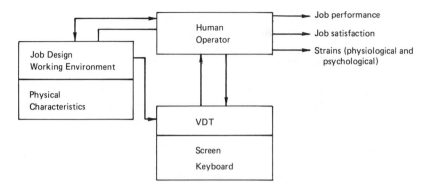

Physical Characteristics
Furniture and equipment design
Lighting (illumination, glare,
    temperature, reflectance)
Humidity
Noise

Human Operator
Physiological status (age, pathology,
    visual functions)
Performance capabilities
Needs and values

Job Design
Task demands (acuity, speed,
    vigilance, workload)
Rewards
Control of job structure and
    pace
Interpersonal interaction

VDT Screen
Regeneration
Luminance (symbols/
    background)
Contrast
Image quality
Phosphor characteristics
Colors
Presence of filter
Symbol characteristics
    (font, size)
Angle of screen with regard
    to operator
Location
Screen separate or attached
    to keyboard

VDT Keyboard
Layout
Type and spacing of keys
Force/travel/size of keys
Angle and height of
    keyboard
Color (e.g., to separate
    function)
Grouping of keys

FIGURE 1.1 Some interacting factors in VDT jobs.

generated, particularly X radiation and radio frequency radiation
in the 15–125 kHz frequency range.

In response to concerns expressed by VDT operators and labor
representatives that radiation emitted by VDTs might be harmful,
field surveys and laboratory studies of radiation emissions from
VDTs have been conducted over the last several years by government agencies in the United States and Europe and by private
organizations and independent groups (see references in Chapter
3). Taken collectively, these studies have examined a wide variety
of models and hundreds of terminals. Measurements of emissions
from older and newer VDT models have not differed significantly.
Measurements have been made both under normal operating
conditions and under conditions designed to maximize

potential emissions (by using maximum contrast and screen brightness, filling the screen completely with characters, using high line voltage, misadjusting service and user controls, causing component failures, etc.). These studies have concluded that the levels of all types of electromagnetic radiation emitted are below existing occupational and environmental health and safety standard limits of exposure. The levels of radiation measured in these studies have generally been orders of magnitude below occupational exposure standards.[3]

In one study (Bureau of Radiological Health, 1981) VDT sets were tested under conditions designed to maximize the emission of X radiation by combining artificially induced worst-case component failures and misadjustment of user and service controls. Under those conditions, 8 of the 125 sets tested exceeded the 0.5 mR/h standard for television receivers, although under normal conditions no X-radiation emissions were detected from any of the sets. Those eight sets represented three models that were subsequently recalled by the manufacturers to be redesigned for compliance with standards or were excluded from the U.S. market.

It is useful to compare the levels of radiation emitted by VDTs to ambient levels of radiation emitted by natural and human-made sources. A person is exposed to greater radiation levels in all parts of the electromagnetic spectrum from ambient sources than from a VDT. The level of ultraviolet (UV) radiation emitted by VDTs has been found to be far lower than that emitted by ordinary fluorescent lights and thousands of times lower than outdoor (sunlight) UV levels. Emissions of visible and infrared radiation from VDTs are less than 1 percent of outdoor levels. Radio frequency radiation is emitted from VDTs at levels comparable to ambient levels generated by radio transmitters in metropolitan areas. The level of X radiation emitted by VDTs is far less than the ambient background level of ionizing radiation from natural sources (i.e., cosmic radiation, terrestrial radiation, and internal radionuclides) to which the general population is exposed.

Standards for occupational exposure to radiation are based on existing knowledge of both acute and long-term biological effects, and they take into consideration the cumulative exposure of workers to various human-made and natural sources of radiation. There is an enormous literature on the biological effects of radiation (reviews are cited in Chapter 3); we found no evidence to suggest that levels of radiation emitted from VDTs might produce harmful effects. As noted above, we did not attempt in

---

[3]In some cases the instruments used to measure some forms of radiation were not sensitive enough to measure emissions substantially below the standard.

this study to evaluate the appropriateness of these standards, an issue with both technical and policy aspects. Neither did we attempt to evaluate issues concerning thresholds for biological effects of low levels of various forms of radiation to which humans are commonly exposed.

Cataracts

Concern about the possibility of radiation hazards from VDTs has been raised in part by anecdotal reports of cataracts (opacities of the lens of the eye) occurring among some VDT workers. Exposure to high levels of ionizing or microwave radiation is known to cause cataracts, and there is some evidence that chronic exposure to high levels of ultraviolet radiation may also cause cataracts. Both laboratory studies of animals and surveys of humans indicate, however, that the levels of radiation required to produce cataracts are thousands to millions of times higher than the levels emitted by VDTs (see Chapter 3).

Some VDT workers will, of course, develop cataracts, since cataracts occur throughout the general population. The causes of most cataracts are not known. Small, inconsequential opacities of the lens are common; as many as 25 percent of normal people may have such congenital or developmental opacities that do not affect vision. Opacities that substantially interfere with vision are much less common but increase in prevalence with age. Some mild opacities may be precursors of senile cataract.

There have been no well-designed studies suggesting an association of VDT work with cataracts or other ocular abnormalities (see Chapter 3). We cannot adequately assess anecdotal claims of cataracts resulting from VDT work because data sufficient to document the claims have not been published. We found no scientifically valid evidence to support the assertion that cataracts with characteristics of those caused by radiation exposure result from VDT work. The ten anecdotal reported cases of cataracts among VDT workers do not suggest an unusual pattern attributable to VDT work: six of the cases appear to be common, minor opacities not interfering with vision, and each of the remaining four cases had known, preexisting pathology or exposure to cataractogenic agents.

Two pilot epidemiological studies that include analyses for cataract were underway at the time this report was written. The National Institute for Occupational Safety and Health (NIOSH) has recently completed a study of VDT workers at the Baltimore Sun (Smith et al., 1982). Preliminary results of this study indicate that the small size and self-selected nature of the study population preclude any assessment of a relationship between VDT use and the development of cataracts (see Chapter 3 and Appendix B). The Mt. Sinai School of Medicine is conducting a larger study for the Newspaper Guild; however, we were unable to obtain sufficient detail about the study design to evaluate it adequately.[*]

The sample size required for useful epidemiological studies of VDT workers depends on the nature of the cataract in question. If careful ocular examinations revealed a specific, unusual form of cataract in a substantial proportion of workers, samples of the size used in the Baltimore Sun or Mt. Sinai studies might be adequate. But larger sample sizes would be required to detect a small increase in prevalence of common cataracts among VDT workers. Exposure to very high levels of some forms of radiation (millions of times higher than levels emitted by VDTs) produces cataracts of characteristic appearance. Similar cataracts (specifically, posterior capsular and cortical cataracts) may, however, occur idiopathically.

The weight of available evidence indicates that an association between VDT work and the development of cataracts is highly improbable. Thus, unless contrary evidence is produced by pilot studies now under way, we believe that large-scale epidemiological studies of cataracts among VDT workers are not now justified.

Field Surveys Based on Self-Reports of VDT Operators

Several studies have been published in which surveys of VDT operator complaints were reported. The findings and conclusions of these surveys and of several experimental studies have been widely cited, especially in nontechnical articles, as evidence that VDT work causes visual problems. Our review of field surveys (see Chapter 2) indicates that existing studies have not established whether VDT work per se produces more visual complaints than comparable non-VDT work. Neither have those studies established the causal factors underlying the complaints of workers regarding visual difficulties.

The methods used in field studies have been heterogeneous (see Table 2.1 in Chapter 2). The surveys have generally used both health questionnaires, with questions on ocular, musculoskeletal, and other physical complaints, and psychological questionnaires with items on psychological states, job satisfaction, and job characteristics. Some surveys have included measurements of

---

[*]Results from the Mt. Sinai study were not available when our report was completed.

visual status, such as acuity and phoria, and some have recorded information on workplace conditions, such as lighting levels and postural constraints of workstations.

The prevalence of visual and musculoskeletal complaints reported by VDT operators has varied greatly among surveys, probably because of the diverse methods used and differences in the populations studied. In some studies, more than one-half of the VDT workers complained of some degree of visual discomfort. When comparison groups have been used, the percentages of non-VDT workers reporting the same symptoms have generally been lower. In most surveys that have used comparison groups, however, the VDT and non-VDT groups have not been matched to control for differences (e.g., in demographic characteristics, workstation design, job design) other than the use of VDTs. Appropriate multivariate statistical procedures have seldom been used in VDT studies. Several of the studies have other flaws in method (such as low response rates or potential bias in selection of respondents) that severely limit the possibility of interpreting apparent differences. Thus it is not possible to determine from existing studies to what extent complaints reported by VDT operators have resulted from the VDT itself as opposed to such factors as workstation or job design.

Video display image characteristics, workstation features such as ambient lighting, and the design of VDT jobs may all affect the visual comfort of workers as well as their performance, job satisfaction, and levels of job-related stress. Extensive, well-designed research would be required to determine the relative contributions of these interacting factors. A careful analysis of job and workstation characteristics (see Chapters 7 and 8) should precede any attempt to design field surveys; in this way appropriate controls can be selected and appropriate questionnaire items can be designed. We suggest that if future surveys are conducted, they should be designed to compare explicitly the relative influences on worker complaints of interacting variables such as job and employee characteristics, workstation design, and display image characteristics.

EQUIPMENT AND WORKSTATION DESIGN

VDT Design and Display Quality

Although well-designed video displays are available, many displays in commercial use employ components similar to those in home television receivers, which can be inexpensively manufactured and purchased. These displays are not specifically designed for prolonged work by operators performing close visual inspection of static alphanumeric characters, often under stressful conditions, in poorly designed working environments. Poor display quality hampers visual performance and probably contributes to the annoyance and discomfort sometimes reported by workers.

Much is known about what is required for good-quality displays (see Chapter 4). Visual performance is affected by a number of display parameters, such as character size, structure, and style, and by image contrast and stability. Television-type VDTs provide less than optimal image quality on several of these parameters. For example, television-type displays generally use medium-short persistence phosphors and a high refresh rate to prevent blurring of moving images. However, these characteristics can cause noticeable flickering of stationary images in VDT applications. Some operators find this flickering annoying, and it may, therefore, lead to reduced performance.

Trade-offs are required in the choice of some display parameters. For example, positive contrast (light characters on a dark background) can help reduce the flicker sensitivity of the eye, but negative contrast (dark characters on a light background) helps reduce the effects of veiling reflections on the display screen and may help reduce problems with quickly adapting to the different luminance levels of the VDT screen and surrounding objects (see discussion in the next section and in Chapter 5).[5]

Techniques for measuring display parameters and evaluating image quality are available and can be used, for example, to give a reproducible measure of the sharpness and clarity of displayed images. Unfortunately, manufacturers have used such techniques only on a limited basis, and they currently use diverse and generally not very useful ways of describing the display characteristics of their products. Because measures of display quality are neither standardized nor offered in manufacturers' specifications, it is extremely difficult for either buyers or manufacturers to compare the quality of different products. It is sometimes difficult for buyers to make informed choices because they are often unaware that data on display quality are available.

---

[5]In this report we follow the U.S. convention of calling light characters on dark background positive contrast and calling dark characters on light background negative contrast. (This is different from the European convention of calling light characters on dark background negative presentation and calling dark characters on light background positive presentation.)

Lighting and Reflections

The results of several field surveys indicate that many VDT operators have reported annoyance with general workplace lighting, glare, and images reflected by the VDT screen (see Chapter 5), and some of the same operators reported ocular discomfort or visual impairment (blurring or flickering of vision and double images) that they attributed to VDT work. However, there has been only fragmentary effort to relate specific workstation lighting conditions quantitatively to the comfort and performance of VDT operators. It is not clear from existing data whether VDT workers on the whole have more problems with lighting than non-VDT workers in comparable job situations. Lighting problems in VDT workplaces are in many ways similar to those encountered in non-VDT workplaces, but some special problems are presented by the VDT (e.g., reflections from the VDT screen). Surveys indicate that lighting conditions in VDT workplaces often do not conform to good illuminating engineering practice.

Many problems related to lighting in VDT workplaces have been caused by the introduction of VDTs into offices in which the lighting was originally designed for traditional desk-top work. The design of most VDTs creates new geometrical relationships between working surfaces and light sources and, unless appropriate modifications in workplace lighting are made, operators may experience problems with glare, images reflected by the VDT screen, and reductions in visibility of the display image. For example, the lighting in most offices is designed on the assumption that workers will perform tasks requiring their line of sight to be depressed 20°-40° from the horizontal. VDT operators, whose line of sight must be at or near horizontal to view the screen, are likely to experience discomfort due to glare caused by this elevation, which brings their point of fixation closer to ceiling luminaires that can act as glare sources.

Because a VDT itself is a light source, operators may encounter difficulty in successively viewing a VDT screen and other direct or indirect light sources having luminances much different from that of the screen. For example, if an operator looks toward a window or luminaire and then looks back toward the screen, several difficulties may occur: discomfort may be caused by the large differences in luminance between the screen and the window or luminaire, and the visibility of the display image may be reduced for several seconds as the visual system adapts from the high luminance of the window or luminaire to the much lower luminance of the VDT screen. This transient adaptation effect may be particularly important when a positive-contrast display (light characters on a dark background) is used.

Losses in visibility due to transient adaptation may also occur when the operator successively views the VDT screen and an indirect light source, such as the source document. The loss in visibility in this case would be greatest when a positive-contrast display is used with a negative-contrast (dark characters on light background) source document, such as a typewritten page. The same type of discomfort and visibility loss may occur when secondary task lighting (e.g., a desk lamp) is used to illuminate the source document. Reduced visibility of display images can also be caused by scattering of light within the eye, which reduces contrast at the retina, or by specular reflections that produce a veil of light (called reflected glare) over the display image. Scattering of light within the eye tends to occur more frequently with increasing age because of age-related changes in the optical media.

Light reflected from the mirrorlike front surface of the VDT screen forms apparent images of nearby or distant objects, such as keyboards, desk tops, or walls. Reflected images of windows or luminaires can produce a veil of light over portions of the screen, reducing contrast and visibility of the display characters. Because reflected images appear to the eye to be located behind the screen, rather than at its surface, the accommodative and convergence systems may fluctuate between reflected images and the display image, resulting in an intermittent or constant blur of the display characters.

No well-designed studies have attempted to relate measures of VDT operator performance to subjective reports of problems with glare and reflections, but studies of lighting problems in non-VDT tasks suggest that they may lead to performance decrements. Studies of the effects of reflected glare on performance in non-VDT tasks have shown that even when the visual discomfort produced by reflected glare is slight, reflected images of the glare source may lead to decreases in performance because they are distracting or annoying. If the reflected image is to the side of and much brighter than the display image, it may elicit a phototropic fixation response in which an operator's eyes move away from the display image toward the reflected image. Phototropic fixation responses can cause a loss in visibility of the display image through transient adaptation effects. Reflected images have also been shown to cause problems with binocular rivalry and binocular fusion in non-VDT tasks.

Differences in task characteristics in VDT jobs might also affect the incidence of complaints related to workplace lighting. For example, operators who spend a large proportion of time viewing the screen (e.g., data acquisition operators) may experience more difficulty with reflected images and screen glare than do data entry operators whose job is typically less screen-intensive. Data entry operators, however, may experience more difficulty with luminance differences among the source document, screen, and background. No well-designed studies have examined incidence of complaints as a function of differences in task characteristics.

Filters can be placed over VDT screens to reduce glare and reflections to some degree. Because their effectiveness is limited, filters should be considered only as a supplement, never as a replacement, for control of light and reflecting sources through proper lighting design. Several types of filters are available, with different levels of effectiveness, at prices ranging from a few dollars to more than $100. Filters are often used without adequate understanding of the trade-offs involved in their use. Some filters, for example, only slightly reduce glare while substantially reducing character image quality or luminance; the net effect of such filters may be to reduce rather than enhance worker comfort and performance.

Human Factors

Several field surveys have reported that many VDT operators experience job-related muscular discomfort (see Chapter 6). Most surveys have been based on subjective reports, but some studies have also included medical observations, measurements of work-station dimensions, or both. Approximately one-half of the surveys have compared the incidence of muscular discomfort in VDT operators with that in workers in non-VDT jobs. Some studies have also compared the incidence of discomfort in specific parts of the body in VDT and non-VDT workers. The results of studies have been conflicting; some have found that VDT operators report more discomfort overall or more in specific parts of the body than do non-VDT workers, and some have found the reverse. Conflicting results appear to be due, in part, to deficiencies in the designs of most studies. The results of one study (Smith et al., 1980; National Institute for Occupational Safety and Health, 1981) suggest that operators in VDT jobs that are characterized by high pressure to perform and low control over the task report more visual and muscular discomfort than do operators whose jobs allow greater autonomy and flexibility. Because of the design of the study, however, its results must be interpreted cautiously (see the discussion of this study in Table 2.1 in Chapter 2 and in Chapter 6).

Although we cannot draw firm conclusions about the comparative types and incidences of job-related muscular discomfort in VDT and non-VDT workers, the results of studies indicate that many VDT operators do experience significant discomfort. It is likely that this discomfort is largely caused by inappropriate workstation design. Video display terminals are often designed and introduced into offices without the application of relevant human factors design principles. In many instances poorly designed VDTs are simply installed at desks formerly used for traditional office work or placed on whatever furniture happens to be available. Operators are often required to work in cramped spaces that leave them little room to place document holders or manuscripts in positions that allow comfortable working postures. Operators in such situations are likely to experience visual discomfort, muscular discomfort, and fatigue.

The physical design and arrangement of workstation components have implications for both visual and postural task requirements. Working at a VDT places a combination of interacting demands on the human visual and musculoskeletal systems that differs from that in traditional office work. The design of many VDTs creates a number of relatively inflexible fixation points for various parts of the body. For example, the keyboard and the screen in many poorly designed VDTs are permanently attached and the angle of the screen is fixed: this configuration allows the operator to assume only a limited number of working postures. If the operator places the VDT at a comfortable viewing distance that allows the display to be easily read, the keyboard may then be at a distance that requires the operator to hold his or her hands, wrists, and arms in uncomfortable positions. This may be particularly difficult for operators with presbyopia (the reduction of visual accommodative power with age, causing the near point of focus to recede). The optical correction for near work routinely provided presbyopic people is likely to be inappropriate for the distances at which VDT screens are usually viewed. Multifocal lenses may not be designed to allow a person to view the screen through the segment for near work without tilting the head at an uncomfortable angle. (The problem is analogous to that of a presbyope with bifocals trying to read labels on grocery store shelves that are above eye level.) Unless multifocal lenses are designed specifically for VDT work, there may be no strategy that a worker can adopt to obtain clear vision without postural discomfort. Of course, this statement applies to many non-VDT jobs and situations.

Static muscle load and consequent postural stress, discomfort, and fatigue created by relatively fixed postures can often be relieved simply by moving the body around. VDT workstations should be designed so that operators can easily change work postures. VDTs that have detachable keyboards, screens that can be tilted to a comfortable viewing angle, and movable document holders allow operators to change postures and aid in preventing postural stress and discomfort. Appropriate supports, such as armrests and wristrests, can also help reduce static muscle load and discomfort.

Although there has been little research on the effects of using adjustable chairs and work tables, their use seems desirable, and there is a great deal of anthropometric data that can be used to design adjustable furniture for different populations. Several manufacturers have recently begun offering adjustable furniture for use with VDTs. Although some of this furniture is well designed, the claims of some manufacturers that their equipment is designed using principles of ergonomics or human factors do not stand up to scientific scrutiny.

Older workers, because of visual changes such as presbyopia and increased glare susceptibility, may be especially vulnerable to problems of poor VDT workstation design. This issue is of special concern in part because the workforce is expected to become distributed toward older ages in the coming decades. Of course, good workstation design facilitates the comfort and performance of all workers.

THE CONCEPT AND STUDY OF "VISUAL FATIGUE"

Surveys of VDT operators have reported that complaints of ocular discomfort and difficulties with vision are fairly common. The complaints have included irritantlike effects (itching, dry, gritty, stinging, or watery eyes), sensations of pain or fatigue involving the eyes, and blurring or other difficulties with vision. Although these surveys suggest that complaints of ocular discomfort are more frequent among VDT workers than among non-VDT workers, it cannot be determined from these studies whether the complaints are related to the VDT itself or to other aspects of the job situation, including workstation, lighting, and job design (see Chapters 2 and 7).

The ocular symptoms reported by VDT workers appear to us to be similar to those reported to clinicians by many people of all ages and many occupations. There has been little effort, however, to interview workers in depth to obtain a detailed characterization of reported symptoms or comparisons of symptoms among VDT and non-VDT workers. It would be useful to know which aspects of visual tasks might contribute to the experience of ocular discomfort sometimes reported by VDT workers and non-VDT workers and how this experience might be affected by the nonvisual features of a work situation. Unfortunately, neither existing VDT studies nor the general scientific literature provides answers to these questions, and the physiological and psychological bases of ocular discomfort cannot be specified.

Ocular complaints of workers have often been discussed in terms of "eyestrain" and "visual fatigue." These terms, however, are vaguely defined and do not correspond to known physiological or clinical conditions.[6] Confusion may result because different discussions of visual fatigue may refer to quite different phenomena: symptoms of ocular discomfort; changes in oculomotor functions, such as accommodation and vergence;[7] or changes in performance of visual tasks, such as reading or visual search.

Several investigators have sought physiological correlates of visual fatigue in VDT workers (see Chapter 7). The hypothesis of most of these studies apparently was that fatigue of oculomotor muscles might underlie sensations of ocular discomfort. The reported effects of several hours of VDT work include transient changes in the near points of accommodation and convergence, resting point of accommodation, so-called accuracy of accommodative response, time required to shift eye fixation and focus between near and far targets, and visual acuity. All of the studies suffer from flaws in method that make their results difficult to interpret (see Chapter 7 and Appendix A). In particular, some studies have not included non-VDT control groups, and others have used non-VDT so-called control groups that differed from the VDT group not only in the use of VDTs but also in many other respects. It is not possible to determine from these studies whether the reported oculomotor changes were specifically related to VDT visual tasks. A few studies have used appropriate controls but suffer from other problems of method or interpretation and can at best be considered preliminary investigations.

The oculomotor changes reported to follow VDT work are consistent with a larger body of research in which such changes are commonly found following periods of performing various near-visual tasks. The relationship of these changes to the subjective experience of ocular discomfort is poorly understood. Many studies have reported recession of the near points of accommodation and convergence following prolonged near-visual work such as reading under difficult conditions or carrying out inspection tasks. Shifts of accommodation toward the resting

---

[6]We suggest that these terms be avoided whenever possible in scientific studies in favor of such terms as ocular discomfort, changes in performance, and change in oculomotor functions that specifically describe the phenomena discussed. When complaints of "visual fatigue" or "eyestrain" are presented in clinical practice or surveys of workers, it is important to attempt to determine more precisely what phenomenon is being described.

[7]See Chapter 7 for discussion of technical terms having to do with oculomotor functions.

point have been found in subjects reading either hard copy or microfiche. Several aspects of eye movements have been shown to change during performance of various near-visual tasks. Some of these changes in eye movements have been shown to be reversed when subjects are aroused or highly motivated, which suggests that either the changes arise in the central nervous system or there is compensation for fatigue of oculomotor muscles. No evidence has been presented to suggest that these temporary oculomotor changes are harmful, although conceivably they might have some effect on performance of VDT and other visual tasks. None of the studies of VDT workers has provided valid evidence of ocular diseases or abnormalities that can be attributed to VDT work.

Several surveys of VDT operators have included tests of such visual functions as acuity, astigmatism, stereopsis, phoria, and color vision. Unfortunately, there has been only limited effort to determine whether the status of these visual functions has any correlation with ocular complaints of VDT workers. There are a number of clinical conditions (especially those involving small uncorrected refractive errors and oculomotor imbalances) that can cause visual difficulties with prolonged near work or critical detail work. It is possible that such conditions might underlie some of the complaints of some VDT workers and non-VDT workers. If so, careful clinical examination of those workers would be important, and appropriate corrective lenses might relieve their symptoms.

The lack of objective measures of ocular discomfort has made it difficult to determine possible causal factors. It is easier to determine what factors influence the visual performance of VDT workers, because performance is more readily measured than discomfort (see Chapter 4). It is often assumed that conditions facilitating effective visual performance are less likely to produce ocular discomfort; however, the complex relationships among visual performance, comfort, and psychological variables have not been thoroughly explored.

It is important to ask whether there are factors in VDT visual tasks that are inherently different from those in comparable non-VDT visual tasks and if so, whether those factors might affect worker comfort and performance. We cannot completely answer this question because there has been only limited analysis of visual and cognitive functions in VDT work tasks. Some unique features of VDTs and VDT work are apparent. For example, the reflection of images by the VDT screen (discussed above), can cause difficulties when no preventive measures are taken. Some other features that are not inherent in VDTs or in VDT work are often arranged in a potentially problematic way (e.g., the positioning of VDT screens at angles or distances that are incompatible with conventional designs of bifocal spectacles, noted above). Many features of VDT visual tasks are, of course, similar to those of visual tasks in non-VDT jobs. It seems likely that with proper design of VDT display characteristics, workplace lighting, workstations, and jobs, VDT work would not cause any unique visual problems (see Chapter 9).

JOB DESIGN AND PSYCHOSOCIAL STRESS

There has been little formal study of psychosocial aspects of work involving video display terminals (see Chapter 8). A few studies have attempted to identify psychosocial stressors in VDT work and to relate them to self-reports of employee well-being and in some cases to physiological changes such as increased blood pressure. Although some studies have found that VDT operators report high levels of job-related stress, no psychosocial stressors or health-related outcomes have been shown to be unique to work involving VDTs. However, the research literature is inconclusive because of problems in the designs of most studies. The data that exist suggest that where negative health effects do appear, they may stem from factors in the job itself (including but not limited to the VDT component) or from organizational relationships involving the employees.

Jobs in which VDTs are used are not purely "VDT jobs," even when the VDT dominates everything else about the job. The total job is defined less by the particular equipment used than by what the equipment is used for: what the worker is expected to produce, the methods and procedures to be followed, the skills and abilities required, and the interactions with other people on the job. It is possible to design jobs carefully so that the work experience is satisfying and productive, but in practice most jobs develop with little real planning, and whatever planning occurs is generally more concerned with the equipment than the person who uses it.

At a public symposium organized by the panel, labor representatives described some VDT jobs that clearly are badly designed; workers in these jobs must perform highly repetitive tasks at a fast pace with no opportunity to vary the structure or pace of the work or even to adjust uncomfortable equipment. Of course, not all VDT jobs are badly designed, but unfortunately, we have no data on what percentage of them are. Existing literature suggests that most complaints are reported by workers in jobs in which a single task (such as data entry) dominates the work day, pay is relatively low, and the workers' responsibility is limited to maintaining output and avoiding errors. Such jobs might be seen as highly undesirable in that they stifle human initiative, creativity, and sense of achievement. The question that demands answering is whether VDT workers who complain of problems are responding to the equipment, the basic nature of the job, or their perceptions of the job and its opportunitites and limitations.

Jobs in which VDTs are used--as well as jobs in which VDTs are not used--vary greatly across factors that may act as sources of psychosocial stress. These sources include the design of the job itself, the social and psychological environment of the workplace, and the broader organizational system of which the worker is a part. One useful approach to analyzing the psychosocial stressors in a work situation is to examine the degree of fit between the characteristics of workers and the characteristics of work situations (see Chapter 8). The assumption underlying this approach is that a lack of fit between the characteristics of worker and work environment leads to strain and poor performance. Two kinds of person-environment fit, which may not always represent two mutually exclusive classifications, can be examined: one is the fit between a worker's needs (or preferences, desires, values, etc.) and the related supplies for these needs in his or her job environment; the other is the fit between a worker's abilities and the demands of his or her job. This person-environment fit approach has not yet been applied to work involving VDTs, but it has been applied to the study of stressors in other work situations, and it can provide a useful conceptual framework in which to study possible psychosocial stressors in VDT work.

For example, VDT jobs, like other jobs, vary greatly on such dimensions as the amount of control given an employee and the employee's opportunity to participate in decisions that affect the way in which his or her work is carried out. VDT jobs vary in the extent to which an employee can control the introduction into the workplace of VDT equipment, the amount of incoming work and associated deadlines, the variety of the work content, the amount and scheduling of time spent at the VDT, and the extent of inter-actions with other people. Although research on VDT use does not permit firm conclusions as to how variations in control influence employee well-being, research on other types of work suggests that lack of control has measurable, undesirable effects on employee well-being. Because individuals vary in their need for control, the person-environment fit approach would predict that lack of (or too much) control can act as a psychosocial stressor for workers in jobs in which there is a misfit between the worker and the job on this dimension.

VDT jobs, like other jobs, also vary in a number of other pos-sible sources of stress, including complexity of the work, quanti-tative workload, predictability of events (such as computer system breakdowns or processing delays), threat of job loss, and social support. This list is not exhaustive, of course, but indicates the range of dimensions on which VDT jobs and other jobs vary and suggests potential stressors that might usefully be studied within the framework of person-environment fit theory. Systematic studies of the relative contribution of each psychosocial stressor as a component of the context in which the VDT is used would provide a much greater increase in knowledge about the psychogenic health effects of VDT use than studies that have simply compared complaints of job-related stress in a "VDT group" and a "non-VDT group" without attempting to match workers and jobs in other respects. These kinds of evaluations would allow the examination of the contributions of the worker and of the VDT and its work environment to employee well-being, and could help generate options for improving the fit between a person and a job.

Most, if not all, psychosocial stressors that may be associated with VDT work under conditions in which the work is not organized with the well-being of the worker in mind do not seem to be inherent to VDT technology and software. VDTs, like any other work technology, can be used properly or improperly, and VDT work can be organized so that it reduces stress and increases productivity or increases stress and reduces productivity.

In many, but not all, job settings, VDTs have been introduced without consultation with the workers who are to use them. The manner in which this new technology is introduced may influence workers' perceptions of the VDT. The private use of VDTs (e.g., home computers and word processors) similar to those used occupationally is growing rapidly. It might be interesting to compare user attitudes in private and industrial settings; there have as yet been no formal studies making such a comparison.

DESIGN, PRACTICE, AND STANDARDS

Principles of Good Design and Practice

VDTs have often been designed and introduced into workplaces with little attention to well-established principles of, and existing data about, good design and practice. There is a large base of knowledge about image quality, workplace design, lighting and reflections, and industrial and organizational psychology that has often been disregarded or inappropriately applied. It is likely that problems with and concerns about the use of VDTs would be greatly alleviated by the appropriate application of this knowledge to the design of VDT equipment and VDT jobs (see Chapter 9).

We strongly urge designers of VDT jobs to draw upon well-established principles for organizing work in ways that are conducive to the well-being of workers (see Chapter 9). Our analysis suggests two principles that should be given special consideration: (1) stress can best be reduced by optimizing the fit between a worker and his or her working environment, rather than standardizing environments regardless of individual needs and abilities; and (2) participation in decision making and some degree of individual control over the nature and pace of work allows workers to achieve maximum person-environment fit. Among the implications of these principles is that flexibility is preferable to fixed rest breaks. It should be noted, however, that rigidly designed jobs with high quotas for productivity, in which the output of workers is monitored moment by moment, allow little or no flexibility; in these cases, fixed rest breaks may provide the only opportunity to move around or to rest tired eyes.

Public Education

To a substantial degree, alleviation of problems associated with the use of VDTs depends on educating users, both those who decide to have others use such equipment and those who operate it. Users of VDTs and of related equipment need to be aware that many ergonomic problems can be overcome immediately by applying what is already known about display quality and workplace design; it is not necessary to wait for further research (see Chapters 6 and 9). Well-designed, high-quality displays and related workplace equipment and furniture are commercially available. Manufacturers should standardize definitions of equipment characteristics and techniques used to measure them and make this information available so that users will be in a position to make informed choices. Users should also learn as much as possible about the characteristics of well-designed equipment so that they can effectively evaluate and compare products. Users can also apply existing knowledge in reducing glare and in adjusting angles of view, visual distances between display and operator, display contrast and luminance, and so on. Both managers and workers can support the use of good employee-management practices in the introduction and use of VDTs.

Education about these matters involves more than just making such information available. Consumers need to learn how to distinguish between reports that are based on scientific research and those that argue from uncontrolled collections of cases. The scientific community could help with this goal by taking a more active stance in contributing information to media that are widely available to the general public (while continuing to document findings through scientific publication). The media could help by reporting both the claims made by various parties regarding the

health effects of VDTs and the <u>basis</u> for those claims; such reporting may require better knowledge of scientific methods on the
part of reporters and writers. Unfortunately, sensationalized
accounts often draw more attention, and sometimes more
credence, than do careful analyses of evidence.

Standards and Guidelines for VDT Use[8]

Standards have been proposed or enacted, primarily in Europe, for
VDT design characteristics and use. Various standards have been
specified in labor agreements, directives or guidelines from government agencies, or legislation. Some standards cover workstation design features, image display characteristics, and lighting
and reflection conditions; some also specify provision of rest
breaks, operator training in VDT use, and eye examinations for
VDT operators. Most, though not all, standards specify numerical
values for such parameters as display character size, luminance
levels, key force, and viewing distance. Substantial differences
and conflicts in specifications are found among these standards,
which appear to be based on varying assumptions (see Chapter 9).
Some specifications do not have a clear empirical basis, and some
do not reflect existing knowledge about visual performance.

Judicious use of guidelines and standards can be helpful, but we
feel that it would be premature to establish mandatory standards.
Careful research and discussion are needed to resolve conflicts in
the specifications given in existing and proposed standards. There
do not appear to have been any careful follow-up studies to
evaluate the efficacy of standards now in use. Because VDT
technology is rapidly evolving, standards that are premature may
impede improvements or become irrelevant. Standardized,
appropriate methods for measuring and evaluating image quality
are needed in order to develop appropriate guidelines for displays.
Without such standard techniques, compliance with mandatory

---

[8]In this discussion we use <u>standards</u> to refer to specifications of
values for design parameters to which strict adherence is
expected. These include legally binding specifications, such as the
German Safety Standards; specifications written into contracts,
such as the U.S. Military Standard 1472C; and specifications
voluntarily adopted by industry, such as those promulgated by the
American National Standards Institute. In contrast we use
<u>guidelines</u> to refer to specifications that are suggested with the
understanding that implementation be flexible, depending on
circumstances and needs.

standards (including those that specify equipment maintenance procedures and schedules) would be difficult.

In addition to careful, systematic research, we suggest that there should be a continuing dialogue among scientists, manufacturers, and VDT users so that useful guidelines can evolve. It seems likely that different sets of guidelines will be appropriate for different kinds of VDT applications and operations.

RESEARCH NEEDS

A number of questions raised in our analysis of the research literature on effects of VDT work remain unanswered. Many of these questions could be answered by appropriately designed research. Chapter 2 discusses criteria that should be considered in the proper design of research. We suggest several avenues of research that might be taken, but we urge that competing priorities in the field of occupational health be carefully considered (Chapter 10).

Objective measures that can be used to relate visual discomfort to patterns of visual activity, VDT characteristics, and visual performance are needed. Such research would be relevant to an understanding of performance of a range of near-work tasks in addition to VDT work. The implications of positive- versus negative-contrast displays should be investigated in greater depth. Research on the efficacy of screen filters is needed to evaluate the claims made by manufacturers. Research comparing cathode-ray tube displays to geometrically stable displays (e.g., gas or electroluminescent panels) would also be useful.

We suggest that research on factors such as workload, social support, and task complexity that affect all jobs--including but not limited to VDT work--be given priority over research with a narrow focus on what is stressful or not stressful about VDT work per se.

2
Critique of Survey Methodology

INTRODUCTION

When society is faced with a proposition that something, usually something new, is potentially harmful, it can take either (or both) of two opposing positions. One position, the null hypothesis, is that the effect (harm) cannot be assumed until there is scientific evidence of it. The other position is that potential harm should be assumed until there is proof that it does not exist. While at first glance the latter position may appear attractive, it presents problems. Demonstrating with absolute certainty that something produces no harm is an impossible task both logically and practically. How many years and dollars should be spent to try to rule out the infinite number of all possibilities for how VDTs--or any technology--might be harmful in order to prove no harm? There are literally hundreds of mental and physical disease categories that would need to be examined specifically by careful scientific analysis. And there would be an almost endless number of properties of VDTs (or other devices) that might have to be studied.

A more practical approach calls on society to suggest acceptable limits regarding certain properties of VDTs and possible health risks. These limits should be specified on the basis of scientifically grounded theory rather than on the basis of intuition. Without such an approach, society would be placed in a position of responding to the advocacy of any group of people who want to ban or regulate something, whether or not there is any valid evidence to justify their concerns. Thus, preliminary findings suggesting harm or assertions of harm should be carefully examined to determine what competing explanations might be possible. For VDTs, as for any thing to be studied, research should be designed to develop and test competing hypotheses about effects: Is there an effect? Is it harmful? What are the causes and mechanisms?

Tests of these hypotheses can be made in many ways. One option is to conduct carefully controlled experiments; some of the research surveyed by the panel has indeed been experimental, and it is reviewed in other sections. Another option is to conduct field surveys; most of the research seems to have followed this option.

Experiments offer undeniable advantages. Using well-designed experiments, one can control competing explanatory variables by randomly assigning people to conditions that vary only on the variable hypothesized to be causal: for example, one could randomly assign people to either data entry or data acquisition work and, within those conditions, to a group either using or not using VDTs.

Most carefully controlled experimental research also has some disadvantages, however. Compared with survey research, the cost of data collection per respondent is high. Special laboratory conditions must be created just to collect the data, and only a limited number of subjects can occupy such facilities at any time. Consequently, large sample data bases cannot be economically generated in terms of time and financial costs.

Another disadvantage is that most carefully controlled research, by the act of establishing the controls, creates an artificial situation that may not generalize to typical working environments. Using college sophomores in a VDT experiment may be convenient, but such research subjects do not worry about the loss of job security through automation, nor do they experience the excitement of meeting a new challenge on the job. They do not find themselves in a changed career situation to which they may be resistant, nor do they have the choices or variety of tasks that might characterize a real job. Consequently, the results may not generalize to people who choose jobs with VDTs over jobs without such technology or to people who are on jobs they have already learned to perform without VDTs--in short, the results of such experiments may not generalize to real people in real jobs.

The survey approach avoids this problem, but it has the disadvantage of being unable fully to control competing causes of effects by randomization. (For general examinations of survey methods, see Rosenberg, 1968; Warwick and Lininger, 1975.) The main advantage of field research is the realism of the phenomena it studies.

SURVEYS OF VDT USERS

The aim of field research on VDT use is to describe unique and nonunique concomitants of the use of video display terminals. The question is whether one can identify visual, perceptual, or other health effects of work in which VDTs are used. When such effects can be described, one needs to determine how much of the effect is uniquely proportional to the level of VDT use and how much is due, alternatively, to some other job, personal, or organizational characteristic that accompanies the use of VDTs.

Some health outcomes do show up in the VDT literature. For example, VDT use is sometimes related to reports of stress or health complaints (including visual or postural problems). The complaints appear more often at the lower job levels; workers at such jobs are also more likely than other workers to report social complaints not directly related to the VDT itself--for example, low staff support, low cohesiveness, or ambiguity in relations with supervisors. Some studies find that visual complaints are more likely to be reported by workers whose work is limited to data entry than by those who may have VDT activity interrupted by work with customers or who work in an interactive mode. When negative health effects of this sort do appear, they usually suggest an alternative hypothesis: that they may be caused by correlated characteristics of the work situation rather than by characteristics of the VDT itself.

Table 2.1 summarizes six studies comparing VDT work to non-VDT work or examining a range of VDT exposure. A critical appraisal of these studies indicates that they are uneven with regard to a number of basic criteria for drawing strong inferences from data (whether experimental or survey).

Table 2.1 does not include studies that examined users of VDTs with no comparison group or with no variation in exposure to VDTs. In studies that lack a comparison group (or some variation between persons in exposure to VDT properties of interest), one has no idea if the level of complaints would be higher or lower than it would be in a group not exposed to VDTs. For example, some studies only ask users of VDTs what bothers them. While this might make interesting casual reading, it is of little scientific value because one does not know if the results would be the same or different for a group of respondents who did not use VDTs. An overview of studies involving comparison groups as well as studies using other approaches--one hesitates to call them designs--can be found in Dainoff (1982).

Adequacy of Theory

The lack of a theory specifying major constructs and the links between them is one of the most critical deficits in the survey research on VDTs. Without such theory, investigation becomes shotgun empiricism, and the risk of wasting effort trying to explain chance findings increases. Without such theory, the choice of stressors to study, the possible mechanisms by which they produce strain, and the possible strain produced becomes an act of intuition, for which science claims no unique talent.

Adequacy of Research Design

Almost all the studies are cross-sectional surveys. Such designs do not allow one to determine what is antecedent and what is consequent in studies of VDT use and well-being. Investments in longitudinal panel designs will be required to make full use of some of the causal structural modeling techniques that have been developed for multivariate nonexperimental studies (see, e.g., Joreskog and Sorbom, 1979).

A good survey design for studying VDTs and well-being should make use of psychological, demographic, and situational controls. Then, if one finds differences in well-being as a function of VDT use, one can take steps to rule out characteristics of the operator, the content of the job, and the social and physical nature of the work setting in case they are confounded in part with VDT use. To consider job content and job setting, one needs an adequate job analysis. To consider individual differences, one needs an adequate assessment of such variables as employee motivation and skills. Such data have rarely been collected in VDT studies to date, especially survey studies of the well-being of VDT workers.

There is a tendency for many survey studies to pigeonhole VDT users and treat VDT work as a dichotomy: either one uses a VDT or one does not. More properly, some investigators view VDT work along a continuum and preserve valuable information about variations among individuals in exposure to VDT work.

The tendency to pigeonhole can also occur in attempting to classify VDT use as either data entry or data acquisition or interactive and so on. Valuable data may be thrown out needlessly by this procedure. For example, in interactive computer work, there may be some value in studying the percentage of each employee's work that is input, retrieval, creative, or noncreative.

Adequacy of Measurement

Some VDT research uses self-report measures of unknown or indeterminate reliability or validity. Studies should use multiple indicators of a condition to increase internal validity. (See Nunnally [1967] for a discussion of measurement theory and the importance of multiple indicators.)

Some VDT research uses vague, open-ended questions about work as the primary source of data. Although such a procedure is

TABLE 2.1   Summary of Selected, Representative Research on Psychosocial Correlates of VDT Use

Citation	Design	Sample	Response Rate	Demographic Controls	Situation Controls
Smith et al. (1980)	Cross-sectional survey	Samples of opportunity: 3 sites with 49-130 VDT subjects per site and 21-93 control subjects per site. Control and VDT operators' jobs were not described, so their task comparability is unknown.	43%-73% (VDT subjects) 23%-44% (control subjects)	Yes	Unknown

Reviewers' Comments and Findings

1. At 1 of the 3 sites in particular, VDT operators reported higher levels of job stresses and health complaints than did the controls.
2. Analyses are not presented on whether these stressors and complaints are statistically related.
3. Multivariate analyses were not conducted to determine if group differences in ill-being disappear when group differences in reported job demands are controlled statistically.
4. The data suggest that VDTs might lead to somatic complaints when there is high pressure to perform and low control over the task. This interaction hypothesis has not been tested statistically (e.g., as an interaction in an analysis of variance).

Smith et al. (1981)	Cross-sectional survey	Samples of opportunity: (a) "professional" VDT operators (reporters, editors, printers). (b) clerical and office workers using VDTs (number for (a) and (b) = 250; separate numbers not	38% for (c); 50% for (a) and (b) combined (separate percentages not reported).	Yes	Unknown

reported). (c) 150
non-VDT clericals
(note: no non-VDT
professionals).

Reviewers' Comments and Findings

1. Clerical VDT operators reported highest levels of job stressors and emotional and somatic complaints; non-VDT clericals and professional clericals were similar. The clerical VDT operators reported the lowest staff support, peer cohesion, and autonomy and the highest work pressure, role ambiguity, and future ambiguity and control by the supervisor. The clerical VDT groups also reported the lowest feelings of involvement in their jobs.

2. No analyses are presented testing the relationship between the job stressors and the emotional strains and health complaints.

3. Multivariate analyses were not conducted to see if the group differences in ill-being would disappear when group differences in reported job demands were controlled statistically.

Johansson and Aronsson (1980) Study I	Cross-sectional survey	Samples of opportunity: 95 subjects with objectively varying percentages of VDT work per week ranging from 0% (n = 15) to > 50% (n = 24) working for Skandia in Sweden.	74%	Yes	Unknown

Reviewers' Comments and Findings

1. 65% of subjects complained about lack of influence over introduction of new computer techniques.

2. > 30% feared skill obsolescence as a result of computerization.

3. 63% thought processing delays by the VDT system should not exceed 5 seconds.

4. Excessive workload and unanticipated system breakdowns were major sources of complaints.

5. Mental strain was higher in the VDT group limited to data entry work than in the group that dealt with customers as well. Data entry work had its work pace directed more by technology than by operator control.

6. Open office space design with its lack of privacy was most associated with mental strain by employees. Subjects were asked which conditions of work produced mental strain. No analyses examined the correlation between reported conditions of work, however, and the strains, so the data are based on attributions of questionable validity (e.g., see Nisbett and Wilson, 1977; Ericsson and Simon, 1980). There were no group differences in mental strain.

TABLE 2.1 *(Continued)*

Citation	Design	Sample	Response Rate	Demographic Controls	Situation Controls
Study II	Quasi-experimental design in field setting with psychological and physiological measures every 4 hours from 0900 through 1600 hours at work and at home.	(a) 11 subjects with > 50% working hours at VDT, 9 of whom did coding mainly (VDT group). (b) 10 persons with < 11% VDT experience (non-VDT group).	Not reported	Yes	Unknown

Reviewers' Comments and Findings   (continued)

7. Subjects with no VDT work showed lower digestive distress symptoms than those with little (1-10% working time) to extensive (50%) work.

8. Multivariate analyses were not conducted to see if group differences in strain disappeared when group differences in perceived job demands were controlled statistically.

9. The study suggests that autonomy, threat to job security, and machine pacing need to be studied as stressors that may appear in some VDT jobs.

Reviewers' Comments and Findings

1. Adrenalin excretion higher during early working hours for VDT than non-VDT group and lower than non-VDT group in the afternoon. Pattern appears to be related to working fast in the morning as a precaution against computer breakdowns in the afternoon. On the other hand, the non-VDT secretarial group often had a buildup of letters in the afternoon that may have contributed to their elevated afternoon values. Adrenalin values were expressed in terms of the percentage of each subject's baseline measured for the same periods on a nonworking day at home. Noradrenalin did not differ by group, nor did heart rate. The VDT group showed higher after-work catecholamine levels as well.

2. Although the VDT group more often reported "being worn out at day's end," no multivariate analyses were conducted to determine if group differences in adrenalin would disappear when controlling for this perception.

3. There were no group differences in other indicators of mood. Unfortunately, perceived control over the work and its pace were not reported despite some outstanding experimental work by the Stockholm group on how this variable relates to adrenal hormone secretions (e.g., Frankenhaeuser and Gardell, 1976).

4. Triglycerides, a risk factor in heart disease, were highest in the VDT group during a standard health exam; cholesterol and blood pressure were not. No data were reported on whether psychosocial measures of work might account for between-group differences in triglycerides.

5. The effect of a 4-hour unanticipated computer breakdown was examined with 6 subjects. The breakdown was associated with elevated adrenalin, systolic and diastolic blood pressure, and heart rate. Indices of irritation, fatigue, feeling rushed, and boredom were also elevated.

| Elias et al. (1980) | Cross-sectional survey | (a) 89 off-line data acquisition operators in banking centers. (b) 81 CRT dialogue operators in a publishing and in a pharmaceutical company. | Not reported | Not mentioned | Unknown |

Reviewers' Comments and Findings

1. Job dissatisfaction and complaints about vision-related symptoms and others were higher in the off-line group.

. . No analyses were conducted to determine if differences in job dissatisfaction or perceptions of task demands accounted for between-group differences in complaints.

3. The circumstantial nature of the evidence is not atypical of the literature.

| Dainoff et al. (1981) | Survey | 90 office workers spending an average of 47% time looking at a VDT screen (range = 0 to 100%) and 31 library cataloguers spending an average of 75% time looking at the screen. | Not reported | Not mentioned | Unknown |

TABLE 2.1 (Continued)

Citation	Design	Sample	Response Rate	Demographic Controls	Situation Controls

Reviewers' Comments and Findings

1. Open-ended interviews asked about the nature of the work and how the person felt about it. The question wordings did not mention any symptoms (e.g., "eyestrain"). Amount of time spent working with a VDT was positively associated with complaining about eyestrain and visual fatigue as well as low VDT lighting. Such complaining was higher in persons who mentioned feeling physical or emotional strain. The mention of these physical or emotional strains, however, was unrelated to the amount of time viewing a VDT. Complaints of job pressures and of general job fatigue were also unrelated to VDT viewing time, even though they were positively related to mentions of physical/emotional strains.

2. The open-ended interview format was intended to elicit the most salient responses that the respondents had in mind. Open-ended questions are useful as survey tools at early stages of hypothesis generation and research design. Such a format is rarely used in full-scale surveys since it can introduce error because of verbal ability, both in terms of desire to be gregarious and in terms of the ability to verbalize perceptions. The two groups being compared differed in both VDT use and occupation in a way that could have selected persons with higher verbal ability into the high-VDT-use job. No measure of verbal ability was obtained.

3. No data were presented on whether or not the coders of the open-ended material did the coding blindly without knowing the group to which each respondent belonged. The investigators, who also conducted the interviews, were the coders.

| Coe et al. (1980) | | 257 VDT operators and 124 nonoperators from 17 firms. Sampling procedure unknown. | Unknown | VDT and non-VDT groups had similar age and sex distributions. Within the VDT groups (input, creative, editing, question and answer), age distributions were similar, but input work was almost all female and question and answer 65% female. These demographic variables were not applied as controls to | See reviewers' comments. |

most analyses where
other differences
associated with VDT
work were found.

Reviewers' Comments and Findings

1. The comparison group is identified by occupation rather than by the task categories used to describe the VDT operators (input, creative, etc.). This is unfortunate, for it precludes a comparison of these types of task work using and not using a VDT.

2. Measurement of technical faults in displays, vision-related symptoms, work breaks, hours of work, visual acuity, and other defects of vision, as well as anthropometric characteristics for VDT work. Anthropometric characteristics not assessed for non-VDT work.

3. No evidence to suggest that VDT work poses a major health problem for operators, even given the uncertain characteristics of the non-VDT comparison group. VDT workers report more fatiguelike effects (hot, heavy, tired, aching eyes) than non-VDT workers but the same amount of irritantlike effects (itchy, dry, gritty, stinging, watery eyes). Both types of symptoms were more likely among full-time than among part-time users of VDTs.

4. Informal, not formal, breaks are associated with low eye fatigue among full-time workers reporting fatigue.

5. The VDT and comparison groups did not differ significantly in job satisfaction, boredom, or frustration.

6. Within the VDT group, persons in editing and in input reported more migraine headaches and headaches than persons in creative and in question-and-answer work. These differences, however, appear to be associated with the large number of females in the editing and input jobs.

7. Blurred vision was reported more often in input and editing than in creative and question and-answer work and more commonly in full-time than in part-time work.

8. Although VDT users had fewer acuity defects than the comparison group, the result is not interpretable because there was no assessment of acuity defects of both groups prior to the start of their respective jobs.

9. VDT workers reported more discomfort because of chairs than the comparison group.

10. In general, there were more differences in symptoms among VDT subgroups than between VDT and non-VDT users.

11. Multivariate analyses were not performed to determine whether the job pressures reported by persons in the editing group were responsible for the migraine headaches and blurred vision in that group. The data need to be more fully analyzed (in all due respect to the investigators, the report was made available to the panel as a preliminary document).

NOTE: Studies were limited to those that compared VDT work with non-VDT work or exerted some forms of statistical control for amount of exposure to VDT work. Studies of VDT workers *only* are omitted.

useful in the early stages of research design to determine the language and range of responses people use in thinking about and describing their jobs, standardized scales should be used in the actual field survey. Standardized and focused questions and response scales are not as dependent on the verbal ability of respondents (the more loquacious respondents providing more content) as are open-ended questions. Standardized and focused questions tap areas of interest to the investigator rather than leaving it up to the respondent to decide what the investigator might think is important. While structured interviewing techniques with standardized scales may put words in the respondent's mouth, such an effect should be constant across different conditions of VDT use (unless one is prepared to argue otherwise on the basis of some compelling theory) and should, therefore, not affect the relative differences in intensity or frequency of response as a function of VDT exposure.

Adequacy of Sampling

Part of a good research design, of course, is the method by which one samples from populations of people and of environments. The samples in most of the studies in Table 2.1 appear to be ill-suited for drawing inferences to broad populations:

1. Diverse populations of employees are sometimes sampled and treated as if they are a similar pool of VDT users (e.g., professional and clerical VDT users in one group) without ascertaining if such pooling is empirically justified.

2. Diverse job environments are pooled (e.g., newsrooms and clerical offices). Measurement of illumination, glare, and other physical features of the workplace and VDT are not controlled for and are even unmentioned, despite their potential contributory role in a study of VDTs and well-being.

3. Comparisons of VDT groups and control or non-VDT groups may be confounded by differences between these groups in employee and job characteristics (see 1 and 2 above).

Another serious problem in surveys of VDT users is the low response rate that occurs in many of the studies (and some studies do not even report response rates). Rates as low as 23 percent raise the possibility that the nonrespondents may be significantly different in key ways from the respondents. For example, if only those VDT users who are the most dissatisfied or experience the most symptoms are motivated to participate, and if this is not taken into account, one may seriously overestimate complaints about VDTs. Similarly, if only the most satisfied VDT users respond, one may seriously underestimate complaints about VDTs. Differences between respondents and nonrespondents in VDT surveys need to be examined, and those differences need to be considered when drawing conclusions from the respondent sample. For example, if one found that younger employees were less likely to respond, one could perform analyses among the remaining respondents in an imputative search for any age differences that might influence the conclusions.

Unanswered Questions

No study we have reviewed has been adequate in meeting the above criteria for good research, and most of the studies have been flawed in several respects. The relationship between the use of VDTs and well-being has yet to be studied in a satisfactory, scientific manner; however, many questions are suggested--if not answered--by the published literature to date. The following is an illustrative, but by no means exhaustive, set of such questions:

1. To what extent are worker complaints (of eyestrain, backaches, emotional strains, etc.) due to pressures to perform or to the degree of worker control over performance? Are those pressures greater for workers who use VDTs compared with those who do not or for those who use them more? Does the use of VDTs introduce a unique interaction of high pressure with low control, adding further to the complaints?

2. To what degree are job stressors, emotional strains, dissatisfaction, and health-related complaints related? Are the relationships stronger or weaker in jobs involving at least some VDT use compared with those that have none? Are the strengths of the relationships different for either the extent or the kinds of VDT use?

3. If various job demands were otherwise equal, would reported complaints be correlated with the level of VDT use?

4. What physical conditions are associated with complaints of workers using VDTs? Are those conditions unique to such workers, or would the same conditions be related to similar complaints if workers were not using VDTs? How much can workers adapt to such conditions?

5. What psychosocial factors are particularly related to the introduction of or the use of VDTs? To what extent are reported worker complaints attributable to VDTs, relative to these correlated factors?

6. Are complaints such as ocular discomfort related to the hours per day of VDT viewing? If so, is the relationship changed by introducing rest periods? If so, should the rest be total visual

rest or a change in visual activity? How frequent, and how long, should such rest periods be?

RESEARCH DESIGN CONSIDERATIONS

A number of criteria should be applied in designing future field or experimental research on effects of working with VDTs (priorities for research are discussed in Chapter 10). It is reasonable, for example, to expect investigators to use multivariate analyses to identify the relative contributions of competing predictors (competing explanations) of symptoms related to vision or to psychosocial demands of work. It is reasonable, on the basis of existing research, to expect investigators to measure a variety of physical parameters of the work setting for every employee, as well as a variety of psychosocial and organizational parameters, so that contributions of each parameter can be examined while statistically controlling the effects of the others. It is reasonable to expect investigators to view VDT work as a continuum rather than as a dichotomy. Rather than artificially dividing employees into VDT and non-VDT groups, investigators should instead make use of the rich range of variance in VDT work that may occur even within a particular VDT group.

Control and Choice in Studies of VDT Physical Parameters

One particular area that merits attention in studies of the physical parameters of VDT work concerns choice. A VDT operator may be exposed to physical condition A (such as a high-contrast display), B (moderate contrast), or C (low contrast), and inferences are drawn about which of these conditions do and do not produce strain. Such a design overlooks the condition of choice; the operator is always assigned to a condition. If, however, individual differences in preference for variety of stimuli are important, then the effect of each physical condition will vary considerably between individuals.

Suppose that one routinely includes a condition in which some participants are allowed choice; that is, subjects can alter the stimulus to their own subjective tastes (vary the independent variable). It is possible that the mere opportunity to exhibit choice will reduce some psychological strains and complaints (see Brehm, 1966). This could be demonstrated by what is called a yoked design. In such a design, the subject in the choice condition varies the stimulus, and this variation is carefully recorded and used to present a schedule of stimulus changes to another subject. The second subject receives the same variety of stimulus change but lacks choice or control. Care would need to be taken to match such subjects in order to demonstrate that the effects of choice were more than the effects of allowing a person to choose the most physiologically fitting stimulus condition.

Practical Considerations

We do not mean to suggest that field studies must be of a perfect design to be of value; designing research always involves compromises, and probably no study will ever be done that will meet all of the criteria for an ideal field study. Many practical difficulties have been and will be encountered in planning and conducting field research on complaints involving VDT use. For example, it is not always possible for an investigator to use rigorous sampling techniques. Often an investigator is allowed into an institution to do research and simply told what population is available for study. Even in that situation, however, it is reasonable to expect an investigator to take the limitation into account in designing the study and analyzing the data. The use of appropriate multivariate analyses to control for the effects of extraneous variables can be particularly difficult in field research. VDT operators work within a complex system in which many varibles interact, probably in complex ways, to affect their well-being. While the use of multivariate techniques is essential to understanding the interplay among the variables, the selection of which varibles and which interactions between variables to study can be problematic because there are scores of such variables and possible interactions. We do not yet have sufficient knowledge about which variables are important and how they may interact.

Another problem involved in the use of multivariate analyses is that they require an investigator to have complete data on each questionnaire item for each subject in the population under study; response rates to questionnaire items are, however, difficult to predict in field research, and what may appear in the design phase to be a substantial population for study may in fact become small in the analysis stage when there are missing data. Absenteeism and job turnover make missing data an especially difficult problem in longitudinal studies.

What is needed at this stage are some studies of samples of convenience that at least attempt to apply variety and detail of measures and in-depth techniques of data analysis. Once such studies are completed, the value of random sample designs (which may be valuable in drawing inferences about the total population of VDT users) can be more reasonably assessed.

3
Radiation Emissions and Their Effects

TYPES AND LEVELS OF RADIATION EMITTED BY VDTS

Most electronic products, including video display terminals, emit electromagnetic radiation. The types and levels of radiation emitted vary with the device. VDTs are designed to emit visible radiation (light), and all electronic products that increase in temperature, including VDTs, emit infrared (thermal) radiation. Electronic products in which certain types of high-voltage components are used can produce X radiation (i.e., X rays). For example, VDTs that use a cathode-ray tube (CRT) display produce internal X radiation; the tube face, however, is designed to filter out this radiation so that it does not leave the tube. CRTs also have sweep oscillator circuits, which emit radio frequency radiation. The radiation emitted in any part of the spectrum may be either broadband (e.g., most infrared radiation emitted by VDTs is broadband) or limited to discrete wavelengths or frequencies, as is most common for radio frequency radiation emitted by CRT circuits.

The radiation emissions of a wide variety of different types of VDTs have been measured, and most types of VDTs in current use have been adequately surveyed for all types of potentially hazardous electromagnetic radiation. In many cases, measurements were undertaken because of concerns expressed by VDT users about potential radiation hazards. Field surveys and laboratory studies have been conducted by government agencies in this country and abroad (Moss et al., 1977; Cox, 1980; Terrana et al., 1980; Bureau of Radiological Health, 1981; National Institute for Occupational Safety and Health, 1981), private organizations (Weiss and Petersen, 1979), and independent groups (Wolbarsht et al., 1980). All of the studies have reached the same conclusion: emissions of all types of electromagnetic radiation--X rays, ultraviolet (UV), visible (light), infrared (IR), and radio frequency (RF) radiation, including microwaves--are well below accepted occupational and environmental health and safety standard limits. The principal studies reported in the literature are summarized in Table 3.1.

Some differences appear in the levels of radiation reported in different studies (see Table 3.1); the largest differences occur between field surveys and laboratory studies. In the field studies reviewed, VDTs and measuring instruments were not shielded from ambient radiation; thus, the readings obtained represent the sum of the VDT emissions and all other sources of radiation present. Furthermore, in some of the field surveys, instruments of limited sensitivity were used and the emissions were very weak, so that the actual emission levels could not be determined; in these cases it could be determined only that the emission levels were less than some value (usually the radiation exposure standard). Under controlled laboratory conditions it is possible to use shielding, special time-averaging techniques, and more sensitive instruments to measure the actual emission levels or to set a much lower limiting value. Thus, the laboratory studies cited in Table 3.1 provide the best measures of actual emissions from VDTs.

Studies of Emission Levels

The 1977 NIOSH Study

The first detailed measurements of radiation emitted by VDTs were made by the National Institute for Occupational Safety and Health (NIOSH) of the U.S. Department of Health, Education, and Welfare (Moss et al., 1977). The measurements were undertaken in response to a request from the Newspaper Guild and the New York Times for an evaluation of possible radiation hazards to which employees working with VDTs might be exposed.

The emissions from three units (Harris 1500A, Incoterm SPD 10/20, and Telco 40) in use at the newspaper facility were measured in the UV, visible, IR, and RF bands. (The Harris and Telco units had been used by two employees who developed cataracts.) Luminance measurements were also made on the Telco and Harris units and on an IBM 3277 unit. Measurements of RF emissions and luminance values were made on an additional 20 units of several models (Harris 1500A, Harris 2200, IBM 3277, and Telco 40). Measurements of X-ray emissions were not made during this survey because previous measurements made by NIOSH and other groups on the same and similar VDT models, some of which were located at the newspaper facility, found no X radiation above background levels.

TABLE 3.1 Maximum Values Reported From Several Radiation Measurement Studies

Radiation Band	Bell Telephone Laboratories (Weiss and Petersen, 1979)	NIOSH (Moss et al., 1977)	Wolbarsht et al. (1980)	Terrana et al. (1980)	HSE/NRPB (Cox, 1980)	NIOSH (1981)	Bureau of Radiological Health (1981)	Representative Standards
X Radiation (100pm)	<0.5 mR/h[a]	—	0.05 μR/h	0.02 mR/h	10 μrem/h	Not detected	Not detected (normal conditions) 2.0 mR/h[b] (worst case)	2.5 mR/h (occupational) OSHA[c] 0.5 mR/h (emission limit) 21 CFR[c] 1020.10
Actinic UVR (200-320 nm)	Not detected	Not detected	0.1 nW/cm² @ 50 cm	—	Not detected	—	—	0.1 μW/cm²(100 nW/cm²) in 8 hours ACGIH[c]
Near-UVR	0.1 μW/cm²	0.002 μW/cm²	0.02 μW/cm² @ 1 cm	—	12.4 μW/cm²	0.65 μW/cm²	5 μW/cm²	1 mW/cm²(1000 μW/cm²) ACGIH
Blue light radiance	—	—	1.4 μW/(cm²-sr)	—	80 μW/(cm²-sr) (total visible)	—	< 1 mW/cm²[a] (total visible)	2 mW/(cm²-sr) ANSI[c] 136 and ACGIH
Visible luminance	—	21 fL	10.7 fL	—	—	40 fL	—	2920 fL = 1.0 × 10⁴ cd/m²
Infrared	—	Not detected	20 μW/cm² @ 1 cm	—	5 μW/cm² (< 1.05 μm) 0.4 mW/cm² (10 μm-3 mm)	—	—	10 mW/cm² (10,000 μW/cm²) ACGIH

RF band (low frequency through microwave)	40 mV/m	Not detected @ 10 cm; 520 V/m[d] at rear surface	5.2 mV/m (10 MHz-10 GHz) 0.23 V/m (1 kHz-10 MHz)	0.2-0.3 V/m (background) 3.6 V/m (at contact) 0.2-0.5 V/m (operator position)	0.5 mW/cm² (300 MHz-18 GHz) <1 W/m² (10 MHz-3 GHz) >300 V/m (10 kHz-220 MHz)	Not detected[d] (10 kHz-100 MHz) 64 V/m @ 5 cm[e] 2 V/m @ 30 cm	61-610 V/m depending on wavelength in the 300 kHz-100 GHz region, ANSI C 95.1 (1982). No standard exists for the region below 300 kHz; however, a standard of 610 V/m is being contemplated by ANSI.
Ultrasound	—	—	—	—	—	68 dB @ 40 kHz	75 dB Acton[f]

NOTE: Unless otherwise noted, all values represent the highest reading from any VDT set tested at any point 5 cm from the surface of the set.

[a] These numbers represent the limit of sensitivity of the instruments used in these field studies. Whatever level of radiation was emitted would have been some value less than this number.

[b] No emissions were detected under normal operating conditions. Under worst-case fault and misadjustment conditions 8 out of 125 sets exceeded the standard and were modified or withdrawn from the market (see the discussion in Chapter 3).

[c] OSHA is the Occupational Safety and Health Administration, U.S. Department of Labor. CFR is the Code of Federal Regulations, U.S. Department of Labor. ACGIH is the American Conference of Governmental Industrial Hygienists, Cincinnati, Ohio. ANSI is the American National Standards Institute, New York.

[d] Apparently erroneous measurements of near E-field strength were recorded from VDT sets in which the flyback transformer was not enclosed in a metal shield (National Institue for Occupational Safety and Health, 1981). If the transformer is not shielded, a strong E field can be detected in the immediate vicinity of the transformer. Spectral analysis shows this E field to be concentrated in the low-frequency region below 300 kHz. It is difficult to measure the true E-field strength accurately at distances of ® 5 cm because the metallic antenna of the field strength meter perturbs the field ("capacitive coupling"). Measurements taken at 30 cm from the VDT screen (where this coupling effect is greatly diminished) have been reported to be on the order of 2 V/m (Bureau of Radiological Health, 1981). Note that no standard has been set for the RF region below 300 kHz because of the very low absorption of RF energy in this region by biological tissues.

[e] Measured from screen face. A reading F 1,000 V/m was obtained 5 cm from the top of the flyback transformer when the shield was removed; the reading was zero with the shield in place.

[f] Acton refers to the voluntary guidelines recommended by W. I. Acton of the United Kingdom; there is no formal standard in the United States for exposure to ultrasound.

Emissions of visible, IR, and RF radiation could not be detected, even when the most sensitive detector scales on the measurement instruments were used. Measured luminance values were less than one percent of the standard of the American Conference of Governmental Industrial Hygienists (ACGIH). No UV radiation below a wavelength of 300 nm was detected. At wavelengths between 300 and 400 nm (UV-A), the maximum measured emission was 1/500,000 of the occupational exposure standards presently recommended by the ACGIH.

Because the values obtained for the emissions of all types of radiation measured were considerably below currently recommended occupational exposure standards, NIOSH concluded that "the VDTs surveyed do not appear capable of producing levels of radiation presenting an occupational ocular radiation hazard" (Moss et al., 1977:14).

The Bell Telephone Laboratories Study

The next widely circulated, published radiation survey was conducted by Weiss and Petersen (1979) for Bell Telephone Laboratories. The 33 VDTs surveyed represented 13 different models used at Bell Telephone Laboratories. Measurements were made across the entire spectrum, although not all units were measured in each band. This study also reviewed the problems associated with accurate measurement of weak emissions.

The only radiation emissions detected were from 1.5 kHz to 1.42 GHz in the RF spectrum, and from 350 nm in the UV to 600 nm in the red part of the visible spectrum. The emissions of RF radiation were 1/100 of the most stringent safety standard in the world, that of Czechoslovakia; emissions of UV were 1/10,000 or less of occupational exposure limits.

Measurements of X radiation emissions were reported for 18 CRT units of 11 different models. Only one unit yielded emissions above background levels: the emissions were caused by a faulty high-voltage power supply, and after the unit was repaired, no further X radiation was detected. Each of the other units surveyed yielded levels that were less than 0.5 mR/h, measured 5 cm from any accessible surface.

A Collaborative Study

In a study reported in 1980 a group of independent investigators from Duke University, the U.S. Army Environmental Hygiene Agency, the University of Washington, and the IBM Corporation performed careful, detailed laboratory measurements of emissions from an IBM Model 3277 VDT (Wolbarsht et al., 1980). RF radiation (including microwave) from 10 kHz to 10 GHz, optical radiation from 200 nm (UV) to 10 μm (far infrared), and X radiation from 5 keV to over 40 keV were measured. Because measurements were performed in a screened laboratory, it was possible to measure very weak emissions that cannot be measured in field surveys.

The emission values for all bands at the tube face and other locations were reported to be from 1/10 to 1/100 of existing safety standards, even under artificially induced overvoltage fault conditions designed to maximize emissions. In many instances, it was difficult to measure emissions because they were below or near background environmental levels. Measurements of RF emissions from black-and-white and color television sets were also made for comparison purposes; the television sets emitted more RF radiation at frequencies of less than 1 MHz and slightly less RF radiation at higher frequencies.[1] This study concluded that there was no radiation hazard associated with emissions from VDTs.

Two European Studies

Terrana and coworkers (1980) measured emissions of RF and X radiation on 13 VDTs of 5 different models used in a newspaper facility and in a commercial firm in Italy. One of the VDT units was also examined under controlled laboratory conditions. Measurements of RF emissions were made in contact with all surfaces, at keyboard level, and at operator position, and all measurements were made with a completely illuminated screen. X radiation was measured by scanning over the screen and all other surfaces, with the screen completely filled with characters. Measurements of X-radiation emissions made by the Enrico Fermi Nuclear Research Centre on an additional 72 units of 9 models are

---

[1]In 1967 national attention was drawn to the emission of X radiation from color television receivers. Some color televisions and some VDTs in use at that time used high-voltage shunt regulators that emitted higher than acceptable levels of X radiation (see Bureau of Radiological Health, 1981:6); the shunt regulators were redesigned to reduce radiation leakage. Solid-state circuitry has now eliminated the use of shunt regulator tubes in color televisions and VDTs, and only the cathode-ray tube (CRT) remains as a potential source of X radiation. As noted above, the face of the CRT is shielded to prevent unacceptable levels of X radiation from passing outward.

also reported by Terrana and coworkers. The emission levels are shown in Table 3.1. This survey concluded: "The values obtained for X-ray and radio-frequency radiation were far lower even than the most restrictive permissible exposure levels established by any agency or government" (Terrana et al., 1980:13).

A radiation survey commissioned by the Health and Safety Executive of the British government and conducted by the National Radiological Protection Board was reported by Cox (1980). Measurements across the entire spectrum were made on more than 200 different types of VDTs in 60 companies. Emission levels were measured at maximum screen luminance with full screen illumination. X-ray emissions were 1/50 of the British emission standard for household electronic products, UV emissions were 1/100 of permissible limits, visible and near infrared emissions were 1/25 and 1/2,000 of applicable limits, and RF intensities were 1/10 of the appropriate standard limit values in most cases. Based on the measured levels of emission and standards for exposure, the study concluded that the "radiation normally emitted from a VDU [a VDT] does not pose a hazard to operators either in the long or short term" (Cox, 1980:31).

The 1981 NIOSH Study

In 1981 NIOSH performed a second set of radiation measurements on VDTs in work settings in three San Francisco-Oakland area newspaper facilities. Of the 530 VDTs in use, 136 units, produced by 6 manufacturers, were surveyed. Based on the results of those measurements (see Table 3.1) and on its previous investigations, NIOSH concluded that "the VDT does not present a radiation hazard to the employees working at or near a terminal" (National Institute for Occupational Safety and Health, 1981:68). The report discussed the danger of obtaining erroneously high RF readings with some RF survey instruments as a result of inductive coupling with the flyback transformer. Early press accounts of such erroneous readings had led to unwarranted concern about a potential hazard from RF emissions. In this study, RF emissions were not detectable.

The Bureau of Radiological Health Study

Because of an increasing number of inquiries from private citizens, union representatives, and government agencies about the possibility of harmful levels of radiation emitted by VDTs, the Bureau of Radiological Health (1981) of the U.S. Department of Health and Human Services recently undertook a comprehensive survey and evaluation of electromagnetic radiation and acoustic emissions from VDTs (see Table 3.1). This survey measured emissions of ionizing (X rays) and nonionizing (UV, visible, IR, and RF) radiation from 34 units representing a cross-section of models of all known manufacturers of VDTs used in the United States. Data on measurements of ionizing radiation emissions from 91 units tested between 1975 and 1980 were included and reanalyzed to provide a more comprehensive analysis for both monochromatic and color units. All units were tested under conditions designed to maximize emissions. Potential sources of emissions were carefully analyzed, and measurements were made under controlled laboratory conditions.

The emission levels of all bands of ionizing and nonionizing radiation were well below current state, federal, and international standards and guidelines for exposure for all 34 of the units tested in this study. Under worst-case conditions (including artificially induced component failures and misadjusted service and user controls), 8 of the 91 units tested for ionizing radiation between 1975 and 1980 exceeded the 0.5 mR/h standard for X-radiation emission for television receivers. Under normal conditions, however, no X radiation was detected from any of the 91 units. The eight sets that exceeded the X-radiation standard represented three models that were either subsequently recalled by the manufacturer for modification to comply with the federal performance standard for television receivers, or were not permitted entry into the U.S. market.[2]

Radiation Safety Standards

There are occupational and environmental safety standards for most types of radiation. For some spectral regions, there is widespread acceptance and confidence in national and international standards (see the last column in Table 3.1); for other spectral regions, only a few guidelines exist. For those forms of radiation for which few guidelines exist, there is generally little demand for standards, either because few people are exposed to such radiation or because there is no general concern that such radiation is hazardous at present levels of occupational or environmental exposure. For example, exposure standards have not been promulgated for RF radiation at wavelengths greater than 10-30 m (i.e., frequencies less than 10-30 mHz) because body absorption

---

[2]Personal communication, William A. Herman, Associate Director, Division of Electronic Products, Bureau of Radiological Health, July 22, 1982.

of radiation at very long wavelengths is far below that occurring at microwave wavelengths; see Guy and Chou (1982) and Schaefer and coworkers (1982) for discussions of absorption characteristics and safety considerations for very long wavelength radiation.

Some public concerns about VDTs may stem from lack of knowledge or misinterpretation of existing studies of radiation emission from VDTs. For example, a booklet prepared for workers by the Ontario Public Service Employees Union (DeMatteo et al., 1981) expresses concern that field surveys reported X-radiation values apparently close to the 0.5 mR/h standard. As noted above, however, field studies do not accurately measure the actual emission levels; laboratory studies indicate that VDT emissions of X radiation are usually orders of magnitude below 0.5 mR/h. The booklet also expressed concern that the X-radiation standard did not consider risks of biological damage other than "fatal radiation-induced cancer." In fact, radiation standards are generally based on all known serious biological effects, both acute and long term, and take into consideration the cumulative exposure of workers to various human-made and natural sources of radiation. The appropriateness of the 0.5 mR/h standard has also been questioned on the grounds that it is designed for television viewers sitting across the room from their sets, and thus the standard would not suffice for operators working close to VDTs on a daily basis. The standard, however, specifically limits emissions 5 cm from the screen, considerably closer than the usual 50 cm-70 cm working distance fom VDTs. The Bureau of Radiological Health (1981) stated that this standard is appropriate for occupational use of VDTs.

For some bands of radiation (e.g., in the UV-B portion of the UV spectrum and the microwave portion of the RF spectrum) it has been suggested that chronic exposure to levels below threshold for acute effects might produce a cumulative effect and over many years lead to the development of cataracts. To our knowledge there have been no studies of chronic exposure to VDTs; however, we again emphasize that the levels of radiation emitted by VDTs are much lower than background levels.

VDT Emissions and Ambient Radiation

The previous sections compared VDT emission levels with occupational and environmental standards. For perspective, VDT radiation emissions should also be compared with exposure to ambient radiation. The sources of ambient, or natural background, radiation are cosmic radiation, terrestrial radiation, and naturally occurring radionuclides deposited in the body primarily from inhalation and ingestion in air, food, and water.

A person is exposed to greater radiation levels in all parts of the spectrum from ambient sources than from a VDT. According to the National Research Council (1980:3), "The major sources of the ionizing radiation to which the general population is exposed continue to be natural background (with a whole-body dose of about 100 mrem/yr) and medical applications of radiation (which contribute similar doses to various tissues of the body)." This level exceeds by far the exposure likely from a typical VDT.

Studies indicate that the level of UV radiation emitted by VDTs is far less than the UV radiation emitted by ordinary fluorescent light that falls on a VDT screen and is reflected. Outdoor UV radiation levels are more than 10,000 times greater than the level of ultraviolet radiation emitted by VDTs (Wolbarsht et al., 1980). The ambient visible and IR environment outdoors is 100 to 1,000 times greater than reported emissions of visible and infrared radiation from VDTs (Wolbarsht et al., 1980). Radio frequency radiation emissions from VDTs, averaged over the 1 kHz to 300 GHz frequency range, have been reported to be of the order of the ambient levels produced in metropolitan areas by radio, television, and communications transmitters (Wolbarsht et al., 1980).

BIOLOGICAL EFFECTS OF RADIATION

A complete review of the adverse health effects of electro-magnetic radiation is clearly beyond the scope of this report; however, this section briefly summarizes the biological effects generally accepted by the scientific community as constituting health hazards, and the final section discusses in some detail the issue of cataracts. In general, the eye is one of the organs most sensitive to injury by most types of radiation emitted by VDTs. The specific effects depend on which structures in the eye absorb significant amounts of radiation; the effects vary with the frequency and wavelength of the incident radiation.

Ionizing Radiation

Few, if any, health hazards have been studied more extensively than those related to exposure to ionizing radiation, including X rays and other types of ionizing radiation. Several reviews of current knowledge concerning the biological effects of ionizing radiation have recently been published, including a report of the National Academy of Sciences (National Research Council, 1980).

VDT workers have expressed concern that exposure to radiation emitted by VDTs might lead to formation of cataracts (the nature and causes of cataracts are discussed below). Available data indicate that the threshold doses for induction of cataracts in humans by X radiation are from 200 to 500 rad for a single exposure and around 1,000 rad for exposure spread over a period of several months (National Research Council, 1980).[3] Dose-response data on human exposure for longer periods have not been reported. In comparison, a VDT worker exposed to 0.01 mR/h would absorb less than 1 rad in 40 years of work at VDTs.[4]

VDT operators have also expressed concern that adverse effects on pregnancy may result from exposure to radiation emitted by VDTs. There have been reports of clusters of spontaneous abortions, miscarriages, and birth defects among VDT operators in four offices in the United States and Canada (Microwave News, 1981). To our knowledge only two of these clusters have been formally studied, one by the Centers for Disease Control (1981) and the other by the U.S. Army Environmental Hygiene Agency (1981). In both cases, VDT work was judged unlikely to be a causal factor, but the reports have not been publicly disseminated.

The level of ionizing radiation generally believed to significantly increase the risk of birth defects in humans is more than 1 rad for acute exposure. For comparison, one may consider that, on the average, people in the United States receive a total dose from natural and human-made sources of about 60 mrad (0.06 rad) during intrauterine life, about 0.2 mrad/d (National Research Council, 1980.) This low dose rate is generally thought not to be a factor in the normal incidence of birth defects. A worker exposed to 0.01 mR/h from a VDT would absorb roughly 14 mrad in 9 months. The report, Biological Effects of Ionizing Radiation (National Research Council, 1980:586), states that "it is impossible on the basis of human studies alone to determine with certainty a dose below which teratologic effects in man are not induced by exposure at sensitive stages in development. Such thresholds do, however, probably exist, and they may be higher for protracted or fractionated radiation than for acute single exposures."

---

[3]The rad is a unit of absorbed dose corresponding to a deposition of 100 ergs/gram of tissue. The roentgen, R, is a unit of exposure dose of X or gamma radiation that would produce ions with 1 electrostatic unit of charge per 0.001293 g of air. For practical purposes 1 R produces about 0.876 rad in tissue.
[4]Assuming 40 hours work per week in close proximity to VDTs, 52 weeks per year.

Nonionizing Radiation

Several comprehensive reviews of the biological effects of
nonionizing radiation have been published in recent years (Acton
and Carson, 1967; International Radiation Protection Association,
1977; National Council on Radiation Protection, 1977; United
Nations Scientific Committee on the Effects of Atomic Radiation, 1977; Parrish et al., 1978; World Health Organization, 1979;
National Research Council, 1980, 1981; Sliney and Wolbarsht,
1980; Williams and Baker, 1980; National Council on Radiation
Protection and Measurements, 1981). These studies cover UV,
visible, IR, and RF radiation.

Ultraviolet Radiation

The health hazards of ultraviolet radiation have been reviewed in
an environmental health criteria document of the World Health
Organization (1979). This report and others (Parrish et al., 1978;
Sliney and Wolbarsht, 1980) note that the UV irradiance necessary
to elicit acute effects is strongly dependent on wavelength; radiation of less than 320 nm is far more hazardous than near-UV
radiation (320 nm to 400 nm). Occupational exposure levels are
less than those required to cause erythema sunburn or photokeratitis. Levels as low as 4 mJ/cm^2 (at 270 nm) have been shown to
produce photokeratitis, although more than 10 J/cm^2 is required
at wavelengths greater than 330 nm (Parrish et al., 1978).

Visible and Infrared Radiation

Ocular effects from visible and near-IR radiation are largely
limited to the retina, where the radiation is focused. Visible
radiation levels required to cause retinal injury are lowest at 440
nm (blue light), the wavelength at which 30 J/cm^2 in one day can
cause a retinal lesion (Sliney and Wolbarsht, 1980; Williams and
Baker, 1980). This level is more than 100 times greater than the
visible radiation emitted by VDTs or television sets (Sliney and
Wolbarsht, 1980). Exposure to infrared radiation in the 700 nm-
1400 nm region at levels approaching 1,000 J/cm^2 (277.8
$mW-h/cm^2$) has caused IR cataracts; however, these levels are
typically found only in foundries and in heavy industries. The IR
radiation emitted by VDTs is no more than 1 mW/cm^2 above
ambient levels. Exposure-limit guidelines for chronic exposure are
typically 10 mW/cm^2 to the eye or for the entire body (see, e.g.,
Sliney and Wolbarsht, 1980).

Radio Frequency Radiation

The level of radiation required to cause microwave cataracts experimentally in animals is generally about 100 mW/cm^2. A previous report of the National Academy of Sciences concluded, "Existing evidence does not suggest that microwave fields of less than 10 mW/cm^2 can induce cataracts" (National Research Council, 1981:3). However, the report did state: "Although there is currently no evidence that long-term human exposure to field intensities around 10 mW/cm^2 can induce cataracts, that possibility cannot be unequivocally excluded on the basis of existing knowledge" (National Research Council, 1981:4).

Teratogenic effects caused by microwave radiation have been reported in experimental animals at levels exceeding 10 mW/cm^2 (Czerski et al., 1974), which is much greater than the measured VDT emission levels in the entire RF range. A World Health Organization (1981) criteria document on microwave and RF fields concluded that human occupational exposure to RF and microwave fields between 0.1 and 1.0 mW/cm^2 incorporated a sufficient safety factor so as not to lead to adverse effects.

Skin Rashes

Several incidents of skin rash (especially face rashes) in VDT operators have been reported in Norway, Sweden, and England (W. C. Olsen, 1981; Nilsen, 1982). Attempts to correlate these generally isolated findings to VDT use have been met with strong criticism since VDTs emit neither chemical contaminants nor any form of radiation that would explain the rashes. Unfortunately, studies have not compared the incidence of skin rash in VDT workers with that in non-VDT workers. Nilsen (1982) argued that the static electric potential that could build up in dry air between an operator's body and a CRT screen would attract airborne particulate contaminants to the skin.

It is possible that under certain conditions airborne contaminants (e.g., fiberglass particles) could be precipitated out of the air onto the skin by electrostatic charge induced in the operator's body, but this has not been demonstrated to occur at VDT workstations. If this effect were to occur, it would probably be most likely to appear as contact dermatitis when an operator touched a CRT screen, where the electrostatic potential difference would be comparatively high. This effect would probably occur only for operators who are very sensitive to whatever airborne contaminants might be in the office. W. C. Olsen (1981) suggested that synthetic fiber carpets not given antistatic treatment (and thus a source of electrostatic charge) might contribute to the occasionally reported incidents of face rashes.

Reported incidents of skin rash have been rare, probably because three conditions would be necessary for such an effect to exist (if it exists at all): dry air to permit charge buildup; presence of airborne contaminants, which would precipitate out on a charged surface; and skin sensitivity to the particulates. The combination of static charge, very low humidity, and the presence of airborne contaminants would presumably be uncommon in most properly designed offices. There is also the possibility of psychosocial stress as a causal factor in skin rashes, as reported by House and coworkers (1979) in chemical industry employees.

VDT USE AND CATARACTS

It has recently been claimed that VDT use causes cataracts (Zaret, 1980a, 1980b). Although no scientific medical study of the issue is yet completed, available data do not support the claim.

Prevalence and Causes of Cataracts

The normal eye contains a crystalline lens that helps focus light on the retina behind it. When the lens contains opacities it is said to be cataractous. Lens opacities involving the central axis of the lens that are sufficient to degrade the optical image and to reduce visual acuity are considered abnormal.

Small, inconsequential opacities in the lens are extremely common; many are probably congenital. As many as 25 percent of the general population may have congenital or developmental lens opacities that do not affect vision (Duke-Elder, 1969). Other minor opacities, often termed precataract, do not in themselves affect vision but are thought to be precursors of senile cataract. These opacities increase in frequency with increasing age: they have been found in 43 percent of people aged 50-64 and 61 percent of those aged 75-85 (Ederer et al., 1981a).

Visually disabling cataracts are far less common. In a sample of nondiabetics in the United States,[5] the prevalence of cataracts that "entirely account for a visual acuity deficit of 6/9 (20/30) or more" has been found to be 1.3 percent in people aged 50-64; aphakia, the result of surgical cataract extraction, is found in an additional 1.4 percent (Ederer et al., 1981a). For people aged 75-85, cataracts were found in 22.6 percent and aphakia in an additional 9.0 percent (Ederer et al., 1981a). Of all people

---

[5] Diabetes mellitus is frequently associated with the development of senile cataract.

with central lens opacities (cataracts), however, less than 7 percent have vision deficits of more than 6/60 (20/200) (Milne and Williamson, 1972).

The causes of most cataracts are not known. Some cataracts are present at birth or develop in early childhood and are usually related to intrauterine infection (e.g., congenital rubella) or inborn errors of metabolism (e.g., galactosemia). Cataracts whose onset is later in life are related to trauma, metabolic and degenerative disorders (e.g., juvenile diabetes, hypoparathyroidism, myotonic dystrophy, high myopia, retrolental fibroplasia), or exposure to cataractogenic agents (e.g., high levels of ionizing or infrared radiation, chronic steroid use, ocular surgery). However, the known causes of cataract account for only a tiny proportion of all cataract cases; the vast majority of visually disabling cataracts are associated with aging (Duke-Elder, 1969). It is thought, but not proven, that age-related changes in glucose metabolism (Caird, 1973; van Heyningen, 1975), chronic exposure to high levels of ultraviolet radiation (or other components) of ambient sunlight (Taylor, 1980), and dietary factors (Chatterjee et al., 1982) may be important in inducing lenticular opacities. The wide variation in cataract rates that are reported from different parts of the world certainly suggests that environmental agents may play a role in their pathogenesis (Sommer, 1977; Zigman et al., 1979; Taylor, 1980).

The Evidence Regarding VDT Use and Cataracts

The Claims

A single investigator has presented two brief reports on a total of 10 patients said to have developed cataracts from the use of VDTs (Zaret, 1980a, 1980b). Neither report has been published in a refereed scientific journal. The 10 cases seem to have been referred to the investigator specifically because they were VDT (or radarscope) operators with lens opacities.

The information given in the two reports is not sufficient adequately to evaluate the clinical conditions of the 10 patients. However, it appears that in 6 of the patients the "cataracts" (termed "incipient" by the investigator) were actually inconsequential opacities that did not appreciably reduce visual acuity. Of the four patients with significant lens opacities:

• One had been a radar technician for 15 years and had required cataract surgery on his right eye long before he had ever used a VDT.

• One, with <u>unilateral</u> nuclear sclerosis[6] at age 53, had had extensive X radiation to her face early in life.

• One had already had one eye removed for retrolental fibroplasia (RLF); the remaining eye, with RLF, high myopia, and previous ocular surgery, had a nuclear sclerotic and posterior capsular cataract.

• One, a 54-year-old with a unilateral "mature" lens, had used a radarscope for 24 years.

In summary, of the 10 anecdotal cases, only 4 had significant lenticular opacities, and each of them had known preexisting disease or exposure to cataractogenic agents.

Zaret has also claimed to have seen a total of 500 people with cataracts due either to exposure to microwaves or to VDT use, but discloses neither the proportion he attributes to VDTs nor any additional details by which his claim can be assessed (Zaret, 1981). He claims that the reported opacities had the typical appearance of radiation cataracts, but the descriptions given do not support the claim. It should be noted that the appearance of radiation cataracts (typically posterior capsular and cortical cataracts[7]) is not pathognomonic.[8] Posterior capsular and cortical cataracts may occur idiopathically without any recognized environmental exposure.

Response to the Claims

The weight of available evidence indicates that an association between VDT use and development of cataracts is highly unlikely:

The 10 cases reported by Zaret (1980a, 1980b) span a wide age-range in which idiopathic cataracts (and insignificant opacities) have been commonly recognized since long before the invention of VDTs. Since many people have lens opacities and many people use VDTs, it is hardly surprising that some VDT users have lens opacities. As VDT use increases, so, inevitably, will the number of people with cataracts who use them.

With regard to Zaret's claim to have seen 500 VDT- or microwave-caused cataracts, even if some of the people had

---

[6]Hardening of the central portion of the lens. In advanced cases, nuclear sclerosis can lead to nuclear cataract.
[7]Donald Pitts, College of Optometry, University of Houston, remarks at the Symposium on Video Display Terminals and Vision of Workers, Washington, D.C., August 20-21, 1981.
[8]David G. Cogan, Chief of Neuroophthalmology, National Eye Institute, personal communication, August 6, 1982.

significant lens opacities and had been chronic VDT users, it would not prove that their cataracts were either associated with or caused by VDTs. Such a claim would require demonstration that those cataracts are of a peculiar, unusual nature or that cataracts occur more frequently in VDT users than in nonusers. One can always collect a subgroup of people with cataracts who also have in common some occupation, avocation, or other attribute.

Short-term experimental studies of animals indicate that the types and levels of radiation emitted by VDTs are highly unlikely to produce cataracts. Studies of accidental or occupational exposure of humans are consistent with this conclusion (see "Biological Effects of Radiation" above). Studies of long-term (years) exposure to radiation of the wavelengths and levels emitted by VDTs have not been done, and few studies of chronic exposure exist for radiation of any wavelength. In two studies of long-term exposures to UV or microwave radiation many orders of magnitude higher than those produced by VDTs, some lens changes were reported with UV radiation in mice (Zigman and Vaughan, 1974), but microwave irradiation of rabbits had no lenticular effect (Ferri and Hagan, 1976). Based on present knowledge and as discussed above, it appears that the radiation emitted by VDTs would be insufficient to cause ocular damage even with prolonged exposure.

Methods of Studying Whether There is a Relationship Between VDT Use and Cataracts

The question is not whether VDT users can also have lens opacities or cataracts, but whether VDT use increases the risk of developing a cataract. (If it did, one would still have to determine whether VDT use actually <u>caused</u> the cataract.) In principle, experimental studies on animals or epidemiological studies or both could be used. In an experimental study, monkeys (whose lenses have radiosensitivity similar to that of humans) might be chronically exposed (for years) to VDTs and examined periodically (with slit lamp and ophthalmoscope and by histologic examination). We believe the value of such a study is dubious, however, given that the effects of radiation have been studied extensively (see above), and levels of radiation many orders of magnitude higher than those emitted by VDTs have been found necessary to produce cataracts. For similar reasons we doubt that extensive epidemiological studies are warranted.

If epidemiological studies are undertaken (two recent pilot studies are discussed below), they must be appropriately designed to be of value. In general, three types of epidemiologic studies can be done to assess the absolute or relative risk of cataracts associated with VDT use (Lilienfeld, 1971; Sommer, 1980): concurrent longitudinal studies, nonconcurrent longitudinal studies, and case-control studies.[9]

Concurrent Longitudinal Study

Two groups of individuals, one randomly assigned to use VDTs and the other not, are followed with periodic examinations for the development of lenticular opacities. In such a study, care must be taken in ensuring that the two groups are as much alike as possible (age, sex, work and home environments, general and ocular health, etc.) to limit the effects of confounding variables. This is the most definitive type of study available, since one knows the baseline status of both groups and can therefore exercise tight control over selection before they are placed at "risk" of developing differential cataract rates. This is the only kind of study that provides true incidence data (the rate at which cataracts develop per unit of population per unit of time, e.g., per 100,000 per year). Its major limitation is the need for long-term follow-up, which delays results and increases costs.

Nonconcurrent Longitudinal ("Cohort") Study

In this form of study, rather than selecting two groups and following them over time, a group of VDT users and a carefully matched group of non-VDT users are examined once and the prevalence of cataracts in the two compared. As the investigator does not know the baseline cataract prevalence preceding VDT exposure and has less control over the selection and matching of the groups, the results are more susceptible to a variety of biases (Hill, 1971; Lilienfeld, 1971; Sommer, 1980). The obvious advantage to this type of study is that one need not follow subjects for years, which reduces costs and provides earlier results.

Both concurrent and nonconcurrent longitudinal studies pose problems: It is generally impractical to randomly assign workers to use or not use VDTs, and one cannot eliminate the possibility of confounding variables (bias) in any matched sample. Although there is no reason to suspect this would be the case, individuals already with, or at higher risk of developing cataracts, might be more likely to seek out (or alternatively, avoid) VDT use. For

---

[9]The terminology used here follows the convention used in epidemiology; for further discussion see Sommer (1980).

example, diabetics might be selected for more sedentary (e.g., VDT) work. Because diabetics are already at increased risk of developing cataracts, a study of this sort might demonstrate that VDT users had a higher rate of cataract development than nonusers, not because users were exposed to VDTs, but because they contained a larger proportion of diabetics.

More generally, a practical, standardized, reproducible method for demonstrating and quantifying the presence of lens opacities is yet to be developed, complicating the diagnosis and comparison of "cataract" rates in population groups. Existing techniques for comparing cataract rates are far from ideal, and have either compared the presence of any opacities, opacities of specified types, or the presence of opacities combined with a reduction in visual acuity of specified amount with or without exclusion of patients with other forms of ocular pathology (Kahn et al., 1977; Ederer et al., 1981a, 1981b; Sommer, 1981).

In addition, choice of an appropriate sample size is complicated by the fact that neither the "background" prevalence or incidence of the various types of lenticular opacities is known nor the magnitude of the risk that VDT use might add to it. Because the background rate of cataracts is expected to be low, the need to prove the absence of significant risk requires use of enormous sample sizes. For example, if one accepts the estimate that 4 percent of non-VDT users have the particular asymptomatic lens opacities of the type claimed for VDT users and decides that a 25 percent increase in risk is "significant" (i.e., an additional 1 percent for a total prevalence of 5 percent), a cross-sectional study requires studying at least 12,000 VDT users and 12,000 (preferably 24,000) well-matched nonusers to disprove a clinically meaningful association with an alpha error (two-tailed) of 0.05 and a beta error (one-tailed) of 0.20. With smaller sample sizes, an alpha or beta error, or both, is increased, and only greater risks of cataract development can be detected.

Only if VDT use produced a specific, unusual form of cataract (such as changes associated with acute exposure to high levels of ionizing radiation) in a large proportion of people might differences in prevalence (and incidence) be detectable in samples of smaller sizes. And to date, there has been nothing unusual in the type of cataract described among VDT users.

Case-Control Study

A third type of epidemiologic study is available that is more economical in terms of sample size. Rather than comparing the rate of lens opacities among VDT users and nonusers, a case-control study compares the rate of VDT use among people with and without lens opacities. Unfortunately, such an approach has severe limitations: it would be difficult to devise a technique for identifying asymptomatic opacities since people do not usually seek medical attention for asymptomatic conditions; and so such a study would, of necessity, be limited to cases of symptomatic cataracts. In addition, selection of appropriate controls is particularly difficult within this study design.

Well-designed longitudinal (prospective and nonprospective) studies could be carried out, but would require careful attention to selection of the study population and large populations; consequently, they would also be very costly. Ideally, several investigations would be performed: by using different groups and multiple controls and looking for dose-related changes in risk, the problems of confounding variables and hidden bias could be largely dealt with.

Two Ongoing Studies

One pilot epidemiological study has recently been completed and another study is presently under way. Both suffer from the potentially biased volunteer nature of the study population and from small sample sizes.

The NIOSH Baltimore Sun Study   The Baltimore Sun VDT study was carried out by NIOSH (Appendix B includes a detailed review of the preliminary results of this study). The study sought to examine the relationship between refractive errors, demographic variables, ergonomic factors, and somatic complaints, as well as the relationship between cataracts and VDT use. Sample size requirements for the cataract analyses were calculated to be 511, assuming a "background" prevalence of 5 percent and a doubling of this rate (to 10 percent) by VDT use. It was recognized, however, that this expected background prevalence and the expected impact of VDT use were both high. The major limitations of the study related to the sample under investigation.[10] Of 588 workers listed on the Newspaper Guild roster, only 283 (48 percent) participated in the full examination. This very high degree of self-selection introduces a large degree of potential bias. Of the participants, 71 percent were current users of VDTs, leaving a

---

[10]Though primarily targeted at local Newspaper Guild members, a small sample of non-guild workers was also included because of a lower-than-expected rate of participation by the guild members.

very small number of controls. In addition, there was no information on previous VDT use by these controls, an important omission if one wished to compare effect of VDT use (presumably a dose-related phenomenon) on cataractogenesis. Because of these limitations, particularly the small and self-selected nature of the study population, the investigators concluded that the study did not permit an assessment of a relationship between VDT use and development of cataracts. Nonetheless, the study does provide some extremely interesting and valuable information on the relationship between somatic complaints and ergonomic factors for which the sample sizes are adequate (see Appendix B).

The Mt. Sinai Study   A second study is being carried out by the Mt. Sinai School of Medicine for the Newspaper Guild. This study has a wider scope and is covering nonophthalmic as well as ophthalmic conditions. The sample size is larger than in the Baltimore Sun study (4,000 workers); it is being done by mailed questionnaires, but consideration is being given to conducting an eye examination on a subsample of the total study population. Until study procedures are final and the composition of the examined group known, it is impossible to predict the degree to which this study will answer the question of cataract risk from VDT use.

Conclusions About Radiation Hazards

The variety and depth of the studies reviewed here represent a comprehensive study of the issues and lead to our conclusion: Present knowledge indicates that the levels of radiation emitted by VDTs are highly unlikely to be hazardous to health.

Perhaps of equal importance, the emission levels from VDTs are far below those emitted by many common electronic products or those present from natural sources in the environment (Smith and Brown, 1971; United Nations Scientific Committee on the Effects of Atomic Radiation, 1977; World Health Organization, 1979; National Research Council, 1980; Sliney and Wolbarsht, 1980). Even if a large number of VDTs were arranged near each other in an office, the summed levels of radiation would be less than ambient levels of radiation from other sources. Although there are differences around the world in standards for occupational and public exposure, by none of the standards would VDT emissions be considered cause for concern (Acton and Carson, 1967; American Conference of Governmental Industrial Hygienists, 1981; National Council on Radiation Protection and Measurements, 1981).

Results from the Mt. Sinai study may suggest whether larger, more definitive studies of cataracts among VDT users are likely to prove productive. Until that time, however, because of the lack of evidence suggesting a real association between VDT use and visually disabling cataract, and the extraordinary size, complexity, and cost of the definitive study needed to disprove the possibility of such an association, it would seem unreasonable and unjustifiable to embark on such studies.

4
Display Characteristics

In this chapter we summarize and evaluate the known relationships between characteristics of video display devices and
observer visual performance, subjective responses, and physiological responses. The chapter is divided into major sections on
CRT display variables, pertinent display measurement techniques
and associated problems, a comparison of flat-panel and CRT
display characteristics, and characteristics and relative effectiveness of filters.

For each of the pertinent display variables, we consider three
categories of effects on human users: physiological effects, the
effects of display variables on measurable and objective performance, and known relationships between display parameters and
subjective estimates of display quality or related physical symptoms. Physiological effects are those in which the display parameter has a known, direct physiological effect on the human visual
or other organic system. Physiological effects typically cannot be
controlled by a user and are not necessarily recognized by a user.
For the second category of effects, representative performance
measures include speed and accuracy of performance. In the third
category, the reported symptoms include subjective estimates of
blurring of characters, headaches, visual fatigue, and musculoskeletal discomfort.

EFFECTS OF CRT DISPLAY VARIABLES

Luminance

Increases in display luminance have several direct effects on
visual physiological and optical responses and visual performance.

Effects on Visual Acuity

In general, increases in display luminance will cause decreases in pupil size, which in turn lead to increases in the optical depth of field and improvement in optical quality. Figure 4.1 illustrates reduction in pupil size as a function of retinal illuminance, assuming a uniformly illuminated retina.

This increase in retinal illuminance, which causes a decrease in pupil diameter, directly affects the visual acuity of the normal healthy eye, as shown in Figure 4.2. While the differences are not very great over the normal display operating range, an increase from approximately 1 or 2 milliLamberts (mL) to about 60 or 70 mL causes an increase in visual acuity of approximately 50 percent. Thus, displays having higher luminance permit an operator to see finer details on the display. The greatest proportional gain in acuity with increasing luminance takes place between approximately 1 and 10 mL.

In general, a positive-contrast display (light characters on a dark background) will have a background luminance of about 1 or 2 mL, and a character luminance of about 25 mL, with a character density of approximately 30 percent. This combination produces a display having an average (adapting) luminance of about 6 or 7 mL. By comparison, a negative-contrast display (dark characters on a light background) will have a background luminance on the order

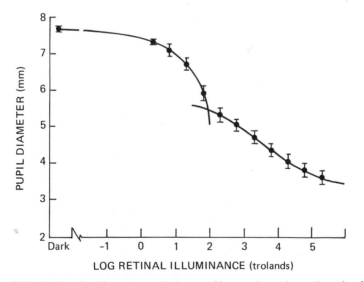

FIGURE 4.1 Diameter of the pupil as a function of retinal illuminance. SOURCE: ten Doesschate and Alpern (1967).

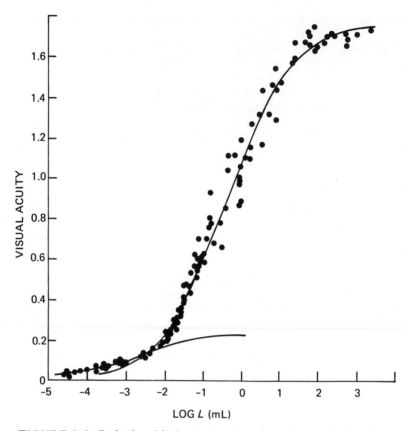

FIGURE 4.2 Relationship between visual acuity and adapting luminance. SOURCE: Hecht (1934).

of 25 mL and a character luminance of about 1 mL, producing an average (adapting) luminance of about 17 mL. Accordingly, one might expect an increase in relative acuity from 1.4 to 1.6, or approximately 15 percent, for a change from positive to negative contrast.

This acuity increase, however, is probably neither important nor real. As suggested by Rupp (1981), the adaptation level is probably not a function of either background luminance or inte-grated luminance, but rather a function of the higher luminance of an irregular surface. Thus, Rupp suggests that the lighter of the two items, either the background or the character, will essentially control the adapting luminance level, thereby negating any effect on pupil size due to positive versus negative contrast. Whether this is actually the case has yet to be demonstrated experimentally for VDTs. There is cause for concern over such generalizations because of the lack of direct application of existing literature to VDTs. For example, there is overwhelming evidence that contrast sensitivity, as well as acuity, increases significantly with increases in overall retinal illuminance (see Figure 4.3); these and other data are based, however, on display fields in which the light and dark elements are approximately equal in area rather than on the unbalanced display typical of a VDT.

It is known that people with poorer eyesight benefit more from increased levels of retinal illumination than do people with normal eyesight (Hopkinson and Collins, 1970). It is also known that maximum acuity is obtained when the surround (the area or surface around the display) is equal in luminance to the display (adapting) luminance (Hopkinson and Collins, 1970). A secondary benefit of higher display luminance is the increase in visual depth of field (based on a fixed diameter of the "blur circle") as the

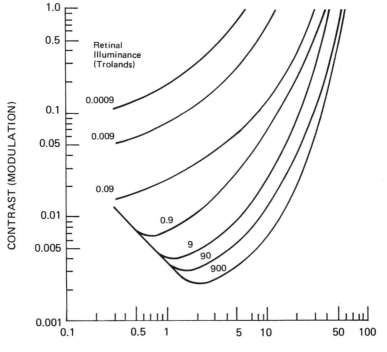

FIGURE 4.3 Effect of retinal illuminance on contrast threshold. SOURCE: van Nes and Bouman (1967).

pupil diameter decreases. Assuming that the luminance to which an observer adapts is in fact the space-average luminance of the display, a negative contrast display (higher space-average luminance) would typically yield a pupil diameter of about 4.5 mm while a positive contrast display (lower space-average luminance) would yield a pupil diameter of about 5.0 mm (see Figure 4.1, above). This difference in pupil diameter corresponds to approximately a 30 percent difference in blur circle diameter (at the 50 percent intensity point), as shown in Figure 4.4.

Again, however, application of these data to VDTs in the workplace should be experimentally verified. As with all lenses, aberrations in the eye are greatest in the periphery of the cornea and the lens. Thus, pupil constriction improves the quality of the image formed on the retina by excluding light that passes through the peripheral portions of the cornea and the lens (i.e., light rays beyond the border of the pupil at its adapted diameter). While pupil constriction is caused by increasing the amount of light in the adapting field, it also occurs synergistically with lens accommodation (focusing) for near objects. Thus, as the eye focuses on closer objects, such as a VDT at a working distance, the pupil will

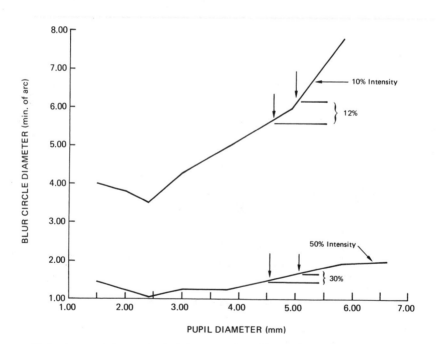

FIGURE 4.4 Blur circle diameter as a function of eye pupil diameter. SOURCE: Campbell and Gubisch (1966).

"automatically" constrict to obtain a somewhat sharper image. Thus, there is a significant interrelationship among display luminance, pupil diameter, blur circle, depth of field, and contrast sensitivity (or acuity). Generally, increases in display luminance will improve visual performance and tend to permit greater cancellation of spherical aberrations by the constricted pupil. On the other hand, positive contrast may tend to make the pupil larger, thereby reducing visual acuity (or contrast sensitivity), increasing the blur circle, and permitting greater spherical aberration.[1]

Effects on Flicker Threshold

Another physiological effect on the visual system resulting from changes in display luminance relates to shifts in the flicker threshold. As illustrated in Figure 4.5, the temporal contrast sensitivity function becomes less sensitive with decreases in retinal illuminance. Thus, as the average (adapting) luminance of a display increases, the eye is more likely to perceive flicker at any particular repetition rate. This effect has been reported in numerous experiments, including those that have included such variables as the wavelength of the light, the wave form of the stimulus, the size and shape of the stimulus, etc. A generalization from the research of de Lange (1958), which illustrates the relationship between the critical flicker frequency and the Fourier spectrum of the time varying stimulus, is shown in Figure 4.5. In general, de Lange found that the Fourier fundamental of the display could be used to predict the modulation at which flicker is perceived, as a function of repetition rate, irrespective of the wave form of the light.

Unfortunately, large-area displays using negative contrast are perceived to flicker at much higher refresh rates than those using positive contrast in a typical VDT environment. Thus, a display with a 50 Hz refresh rate that is just at threshold for flicker at 10 cd/m^2 will flicker very noticeably if luminance is increased to 100 cd/m^2. This effect is in conformance with the well-established Ferry-Porter Law, which suggests that the highest frequency at which flicker is perceived increases linearly with the logarithm of the adapting luminance, or by approximately 10 Hz for each tenfold increase in luminance. The data of Bauer and Cavonius (1980) clearly support this result. Bauer and Cavonius recommend

---

[1]See also the discussion in Chapter 7 of the relationship between pupil size and accommodation in studies of fatigue.

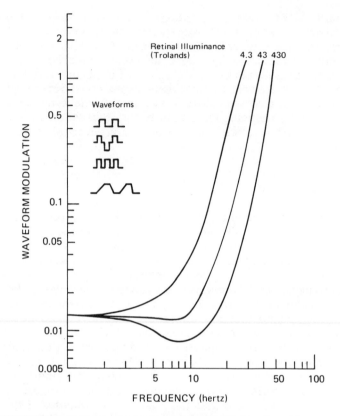

FIGURE 4.5 Temporal contrast sensitivity function.
SOURCE: de Lange (1958). Reprinted with permission
of the Optical Society of America.

a repetition rate of 100 Hz for VDTs with negative contrast. This
recommendation appears to be reasonable and probably indicates
the main reason that manufacturers have been reluctant to use
negative-contrast displays in the past: standard television
monitors cannot produce that repetition rate.

Effects on Visual Task Performance

The effect of display luminance on visual task performance has
been investigated in a few studies. Snyder and Taylor (1979)
demonstrated that increases in character luminance caused
significant increases in individual character legibility in several

different viewing tasks. Unfortunately, in that particular experiment, the background luminance level was held constant, and therefore the character luminance was totally confounded with the contrast of the displayed image. Supporting evidence, however, for the effect of display luminance on performance is offered by Bauer and Cavonius (1980), who found that a higher-luminance negative-contrast display yielded both greater subjective preference and improved visual performance than a lower-luminance negative-contrast display. Further research on the subject of the effect of display luminance when separated from the influence of contrast and contrast polarity is needed, however, before this issue can be directly resolved.

Luminance Uniformity

There is very little research in the literature to provide information on the minimum requirements for the uniformity of visual displays. No studies are known to provide either thresholds of detection or tolerance limits for large-area nonuniformities. In general, we simply do not know how much large-area nonuniformity is a reasonable design goal.

The case for small-area nonuniformity is similar. Unless one applies basic sine-wave sensitivity data to a given form of small-area nonuniformity distribution and attempts to predict the detectability of nonuniformity, there is currently not even a suggested means for evaluation.

Except for an initial study by Riley and Barbato (1978), there is little knowledge of the effects of line errors (on or off) or of element errors (on or off) on display legibility and utility. Research efforts to fill these data gaps are obviously needed.

Contrast and Contrast Polarity

As suggested in the preceding discussion, increases in contrast have been shown to produce significant increases in visual task performance. In addition to the study of Snyder and Taylor, Shurtleff (1982) also demonstrated increases in legibility as a result of increases in character/background contrast. Further, negative-contrast displays have been found to yield greater legibility than positive-contrast displays (Bauer and Cavonius, 1980; Radl, 1980). These studies should, however, be viewed carefully, because changes in polarity were also combined with changes in ambient illumination and absolute contrast magnitude. Again, further research is indicated to achieve a complete understanding of the relationship between display image contrast and the performance of typical workers. In the experiments to date, all the observers used have been young and have had healthy eyes. Since VDT workers often include older workers and workers having some visually limited capability, it is particularly critical that research be conducted with stratified subject populations that include those people representative of typical VDT workers.

No physiological effects are known to be pertinent to the variables of contrast or contrast polarity. Further, the only subjective preference data dealing with these variables has been reported by Radl (1980) and by Bauer and Cavonius (1980), who reported a significant preference for the negative-contrast (black on white) display among the several combinations investigated. Whether this preference would exist under other display and illuminance conditions is unknown.

Raster Structure

Most VDTs produce characters known as in-raster characters. A CRT creates these characters by drawing horizontal lines (scan lines) on the screen. The electron beam that draws these scan lines is turned on or off as required to produce line segments of symbols and characters on the screen. The collection of scan lines is called a raster, and the characters produced within the raster are in-raster characters. Figure 4.6 shows an example of characters produced in this fashion.

Stroke characters are those that are produced by a continuous line process so that they do not appear to be composed of a collection of dots. The printing on this page is example of stroke characters. Note that the in-raster characters shown in the right portion of Figure 4.6 appear continuous because of the close spacing of the scan lines and proper adjustment of the scan line width. In general, stroke-written characters are preferable to characters having a visible dot or element structure. As the spacing between dots or elements increases, the reading time and reading difficulty increase. As Figure 4.7 indicates, reductions in the space between individual dots reduce reading time, and extrapolation of this function to the zero value on the abscissa suggests an adjusted reading time of zero seconds; that is, zero space between dots (i.e., a stroke-written character) causes no elevation in reading time, which is otherwise the result of space between the dots.

It must be recognized that most word processing and data processing displays today use either dot-matrix or raster-written characters, either of which can have visible spacing in the vertical dimension and, in the case of dot-matrix characters, also in

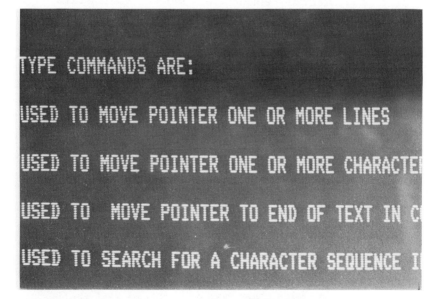

request copies of this report from
ory. Additional copies may be purchased

National Technical Information Servi
5285 Port Royal Road
Springfield, Virginia 22161

ment agencies and their contractor
nter should direct requests for copies of

Defense Technical Information Center
Attn: DTIC DDA-2
Cameron Station

TYPE COMMANDS ARE:

USED TO MOVE POINTER ONE OR MORE LINES

USED TO MOVE POINTER ONE OR MORE CHARACTE

USED TO MOVE POINTER TO END OF TEXT IN C

USED TO SEARCH FOR A CHARACTER SEQUENCE I

FIGURE 4.6 Characters produced on a VDT screen from a raster
structure.

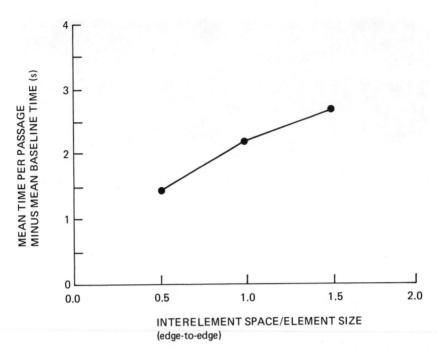

FIGURE 4.7 Effect of element size to element spacing ratio on reading time. SOURCE: Snyder and Maddox (1978).

the horizontal dimension. To the extent that such spaces are visible, reading performance is reduced.

There is also some evidence that dot-matrix characters result in different information processing techniques than stroke-written characters. This is inferred from differences in visually evoked responses of an electroencephalogram recording (O'Donnell et al., 1976).

The dot spacing for raster displays depends on the size of the scanning spot and on the raster pitch. Raster pitch is caused because the horizontal scan lines making up the raster are not exactly horizontal but rather are slightly sloping. Pitch is created so that when the electron scanning beam is rapidly returned to the other side of the CRT screen to begin another line scan it starts slightly lower. This concept of pitch is similar to that used for describing the characteristics of threads for nuts and bolts: it essentially refers to the scan line spacing for VDTs. If the scan line spacing is equal to the spot size of the scanning beam, then the spots making up the characters will partially overlap, producing almost strokelike characters. The more scan lines used to make up a character, the better the performance achieved, as shown in Figures 4.8 and 4.9.

A 525-line raster display will typically present visible spaces between raster lines, which cause character line or dot visibility. A well-designed display having 729 or 1,029 lines is likely to have raster lines that are less visible, and a number of such high-quality displays are currently on the market in word processing and data processing systems. These displays can be expected to make possible performance improvements like those shown in Figures 4.8 and 4.9.

Any visible raster structure is undesirable. Studies have shown that a visible raster (modulation in excess of 10 percent) is detrimental to legibility of either alphanumeric characters or cultural objects. Various means can be used to reduce the raster modulation, and one or more should always be used to eliminate visible raster or dot structure. Among the techniques to reduce raster

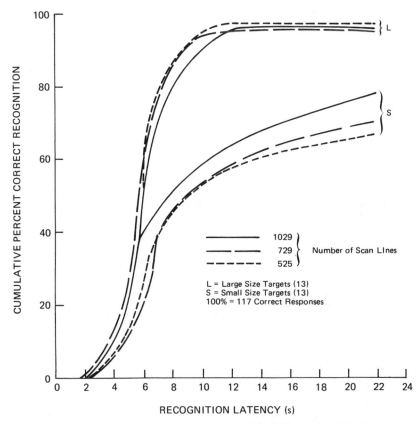

FIGURE 4.8 Recognition latency for 525, 729, and 1,029 line television systems. SOURCE: Humes and Bauerschmidt (1968).

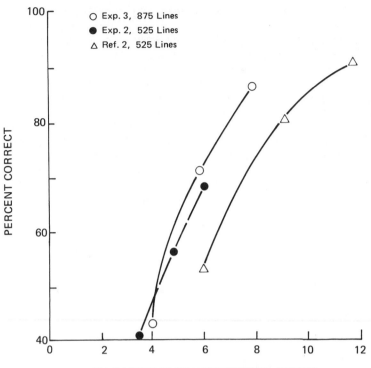

FIGURE 4.9 Effects of display raster lines and number of raster lines intersecting target on symbol recognition. SOURCE: Erickson et al. (1968).

visibility that have been studied to date are spot wobble (Beamon and Snyder, 1980) and matching of the scanning spot size to the raster pitch. It is preferable to select a spot size in the dimension perpendicular to the raster such that the spot size and raster pitch are compatible to produce a visually flat field, that is, a field having no visible raster modulation. In all too many cases, the spot size is too small for the raster pitch, resulting in a visible raster and therefore a static noise source to the visual system. Increasing the number of lines or increasing the spot size in the dimension perpendicular to the raster are appropriate solutions and both result in improved legibility.

Resolution

The resolution of a VDT display refers, conventionally, to the number of elements (dots) or the number of raster lines with which each character is written. It is often also used to include the visual separation of these elements or the number of elements per unit distance on the display. Thus, the term resolution has a variety of meanings, some of which are not well understood or consistently defined.

Assuming, in the more traditional case, that resolution refers to the number of resolvable elements per unit distance on the display, there is no known effect of resolution on the eye as measured by any physiological response. The existing data do, however, clearly support an increase in performance with increases in resolution. For example, Erickson and coworkers (1968) have shown that an increase in the number of raster lines used to write each character causes an increase in legibility. That is, 5 raster lines used to write a given character produce poorer performance than do 7 lines or 10 lines. Based on the results of several experiments conducted by Erickson and coworkers, it appears that in order to reach reasonable legibility performance on a television-type display, a minimum of 7 raster lines is desirable (Erickson et al., 1968).

Using a dot-matrix display format, Snyder and Maddox (1978) found that increases in character legibility can be achieved when the number of dots in the matrix writing each character is increased from 5 x 7 to 7 x 9 and from 7 x 9 to 9 x 11. Thus, the highest legibility level is achieved with a 9 x 11 dot matrix, which would be equivalent to Erickson's 11-line raster. Only slightly inferior performance is achieved with 9 raster lines, or equivalently, a 7 x 9 dot-matrix character. Anecdotal evidence also supports this contention.

There are no known subjective preference effects for various character matrix sizes or numbers of raster lines with which individual characters are written.

Jitter and Temporal Instability

The simple concept of display jitter has seldom been quantitatively addressed. Jitter is the time-based variation of position of displayed symbols due to improper or insufficient video deflection voltages (currents). Some manufacturers specify jitter in terms of motion limits using linear dimension units (inches, millimeters) or percent of display diagonal. Fellmann and coworkers (1981) described a procedure for assessing jitter by focusing a micro-photometer on the middle of the "leg" of a letter and recording the luminance variation as a function of time. They noted that a jitter specification in terms of change in luminance versus mean luminance could be used but chose to offer only qualitative assessment based on the recorded graphs. The Electronics Industries Association (1957) does not address the problem of measuring jitter in its published standards (EIA RS-170) pertaining to CRT display measurement. A procedure to measure jitter should be developed and acceptable limits determined.

Refresh Rate and Persistence

As described above in the section "Luminance," the average luminance of the display can significantly influence the perception of flicker of the display. To combat the tendency to perceive flicker at higher display luminance levels, increases in refresh rate are often necessary. In general, the frequency at which flicker will be perceived will range from approximately 30 Hz to as high as 100 Hz, depending on the temporal modulation of the location of the image in the visual field and the average luminance of the display.

Flicker is of particular concern from a physiological standpoint because of its occasionally reported ability to photically induce epileptogenic seizures. Careful analysis and several research studies in this area have clearly demonstrated, however, that persons who are sensitive to epileptogenic seizures caused by flickering displays have induced seizures only when the display refresh rate is extremely low, typically in the 8 to 14 Hz region, the typical alpha frequency region. Since most refreshed VDT displays have a minimum refresh rate of 30 Hz (assuming an interlaced display), there appears to be no significant problem of this nature induced by most existing video displays.

Of greater general interest is the lack of any demonstrated relationship between visual task performance and apparent flicker at commonly used refresh rates. Although annoyance, headaches, and other negative subjective responses to flickering displays are often reported, it has yet to be demonstrated that a significant deterioration in visual task performance (except as a secondary effect of negative subjective responses) results from perceived flicker. Thus, it is obvious that displays should be designed to avoid any perceivable flicker; however, this is more a matter of operator comfort than one of demonstrable deterioration of visual task performance.

Research recently reported by Grandjean and coworkers (1981) has shown a correlation between the subjectively related quality of displays and the oscillation index, a measure dealing with the temporal variability of display luminance at frequencies within and well above perceived flicker rates. Displays demonstrated to have significant temporal modulation well above 100 Hz have been shown to cause subjectively poorer ratings of visual quality. However, since the oscillation index is computed on the basis of the Fourier fundamental and its first 20 harmonics, over which the Fourier coefficients are summed, it is not clear from this research which harmonics contribute most to the perception of image quality. Furthermore, other characteristics of the displays are confounded with the oscillation index measure because of the very nature of display design parameters, and the evidence is therefore merely indicative rather than conclusive.

Color

Most VDTs use either a white or a green phosphor, although some displays using a white phosphor contain a color filter to change the apparent chromaticity of the display image. Thus, orange or yellow displays have those hues due to the filter rather than to the intrinsic emission of a phosphor. For the most part, the color of the phosphor, all other characteristics being equal, will have no influence on most physiological measures, such as contrast sensitivity or acuity (Watanabe et al., 1968). In general, for foveally fixated images of the VDT-type, the contrast sensitivity is controlled by the displayed luminance (or adapting luminance) rather than by the chromaticity of that luminance, assuming adequate focusing of the image on the retina.

The chromaticity of the image does, however, affect the apparent brightness of the image. Booker (1981) and Costanza (1981) have demonstrated that the red and blue portions of the spectrum are perceived to be brighter at equal luminance than either the green portions or achromatic displayed images. Whether this difference in perceived brightness is related to visual task performance has yet to be demonstrated. There is concern, of course, with displays using the blue or red ends of the spectrum because of the chromatic aberration of the eye: that is, multi-colored displays will cause the red and blue ends of the spectrum to be less accurately focused than green or achromatic displayed images because of the chromatic aberration of the optical portions of the eye.

There are no known performance differences associated with differences in the color of the phosphor used. Attempts to measure any performance differences have consistently resulted in no differences, as long as the blue and red extreme ends of the spectrum are not considered. Further, differences between achromatic and green phosphors are totally subjective, and users' preferences for either are reported approximately equally often.

Reflection Characteristics

Reflections of ambient lighting by a VDT screen can cause a significant loss of character contrast. Two distinctly different types of reflections may occur: <u>specular</u> (mirrorlike) reflection from the front glass surface of a CRT and <u>diffuse</u> (non-mirrorlike) scattering of incident light from the phosphor surface of a CRT. Specular reflection results in the formation of an image of the source that is causing the reflection; diffuse reflection does not. Specular and diffuse reflections from a VDT screen are illustrated in Figure 4.10. There are many techniques that can be applied to VDT screen construction that can reduce the susceptibility of the screen to reflections of ambient light sources; they are discussed below in the section "Filters for VDTs" (other techniques for reducing reflections are discussed in Chapter 9).

Three different VDT screens were measured to determine the specular and diffuse reflection coefficients (see the section below, "Display Measurement Techniques," for details). The measurements are shown in Table 4.1. The specular reflection coefficients were determined by dividing the luminance of the reflected image

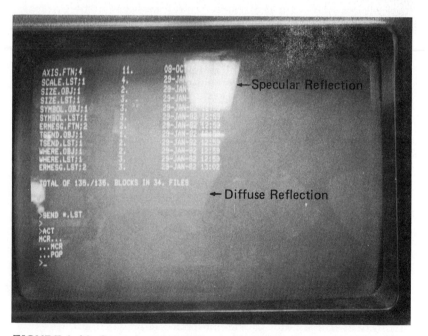

FIGURE 4.10 Specular and diffuse reflections on a typical VDT screen.

TABLE 4.1   VDT Screen Specular and Diffuse Reflection
Coefficients

VDT	Specular Coefficient	Diffuse Coefficient (cd/m²/lux)
1	0.072	0.091
2	0.042	0.040
3	0.017	0.023

by the luminance of the light source causing the reflection. This
unitless number indicates how susceptible the VDT screen is to
specular reflections from ambient light sources. The smaller the
number the lower the luminance of the specular reflection from
any given source. Therefore, smaller values indicate that the
contrast loss is not as great. The diffuse reflection is a somewhat
different entity. It was determined by dividing the luminance of
the VDT screen (with no characters displayed) by the illumination
falling on the surface of the screen. The result is a number with
units of candelas per meter squared per lux of incident light.
Although the units are somewhat awkward, the result indicates
how much veiling VDT screen luminance can be expected from
light falling on the surface. Again, the smaller the number the
better the VDT screen.

A secondary effect of specular reflections is that they result in
an image of the reflecting source. This virtual image appears to
be located behind the VDT screen at a depth that depends on the
curvature of the screen and the distance from the screen to the
source of the reflection; the significance of this effect is
discussed in Chapter 5.

The performance, physiological, and subjective effects of
reflections are the same as those discussed in the section
"Contrast and Contrast Polarity," above.

A Summary Measure: Modulation Transfer Function

The modulation transfer function (MTF) is probably the most
important parameter associated with image quality.[2] Depending

_____
[2]There have been a number of theoretical attempts to develop
measures of image sharpness that can be related to visual
perception. The modulation transfer function is one such measure;
another is acutance.

on the technique used to measure MTF, it directly or indirectly includes the characteristics of contrast, resolution, reflectance coefficients plus ambient lighting, and jitter. The MTF describes the amount of signal output that can be achieved for a specific signal input as a function of spatial frequency. For VDTs it describes the contrast obtainable on the CRT as a function of spatial frequency, which directly relates to the sharpness or crispness of the alphanumeric image.

Many techniques have been developed to measure the MTF of displays (Schade, 1948; Snyder, 1974; Bedell, 1975; Task and Verona, 1976). Each of them makes certain assumptions about the characteristics of the CRT and its associated drive electronics. The most important, and usually the most violated, assumption is that the CRT system is linear. In rigorous mathematical treatment, the concept of the MTF exists only for continuous, linear systems and not for systems in which those conditions are not met. Since the input signal level of the CRT is not linearly related to the output luminance level, CRTs are generally nonlinear devices. When used in a VDT, however, in which only two luminance levels are used (off and on), the CRT operating curve (voltage in versus luminance out) consists of only two points. The CRT used in a VDT can therefore be thought of as a linear device with an operating curve that is a straight line connecting those two points. With this in mind, the concept of the MTF can be readily applied. To achieve the most realistic measurement results, the MTF should be measured directly, without normalizing the function at some arbitrary, low spatial frequency (Snyder, 1974; Task and Verona, 1976).

It should also be noted that the MTF describes the image generation capability only along the direction of TV scan lines. Since the image is discontinuous in the direction perpendicular to the scan lines, an MTF for this direction does not rigorously exist. (The scan line spacing and line profile luminance distribution determine the quality of the display in this direction.)

When the MTF is measured by only one of the direct-measure techniques (Schade, 1948; Snyder, 1974; Task and Verona, 1976) under the identical illumination conditions in which a VDT will be used, it includes image degradation due to diffuse and specular reflections from ambient light sources. It is, however, possible to measure the MTF of the VDT in a dark room and accurately predict the MTF that will result under any ambient condition if the diffuse and specular reflection coefficients of the display are known. If the VDT uses a monochrome enhancement filter, the chromatic distribution of both the ambient light sources and the CRT must be known, as well as the spectral transmittance characteristics of the filter. (Reflections and the effects of various enhancement filters are discussed further in Chapter 5.)

The theory and concept of the MTF have been widely accepted; the methods by which it is measured, however, and the ways in which it is applied vary considerably. A concept similar to the MTF, the contrast sensitivity function (CSF), has evolved for vision (DePalma and Lowry, 1962; Campbell and Robson, 1968). The CSF is often erroneously referred to as the MTF of the eye (Roufs and Bouma, 1980). The CSF is the reciprocal of the contrast threshold function (CTF) of the visual system, which is a measure of the threshold contrast required to resolve a sinusoidal grating as a function of spatial frequency.

For determining the relative merit of the MTF of a VDT, the CTF is probably a more appropriate function than the CSF for providing a direct comparison. If the MTF of a VDT is relatively high (> 0.95) throughout the entire range of spatial frequencies to which the eye is sensitive (0 to 60 cycles/degree), the display should be essentially indistinguishable from the ideal alphanumeric character. In fact, this area between the CTF of the visual system and the MTF of the display is the unified image quality parameter that is designated as the modulation transfer function area (MTFA) (Borough et al., 1967; Snyder, 1974). An MTF greater than 0.95 is typically not technologically feasible in practical VDT applications.

In general, lower MTFs result in a lower image quality, but this reduction in perceived quality is not linear with spatial frequency (Carlson and Cohen, 1978). The relationship between the MTF and ocular discomfort sometimes associated with long-term viewing of video displays has not been explored. Since the effect of a poor MTF is to produce a blurred or low contrast image, or both, on the retina, it is reasonable to assume that if the image is sufficiently blurred, the eye will try to adjust its accommodation in an attempt to minimize the blur. This might lead to accommodative fatigue and visual complaints; however, no evidence for this has been presented (see Chapter 7). How poor an MTF would have to be to produce such an effect is unknown.

DISPLAY MEASUREMENT: TECHNIQUES AND PROBLEMS

Photometric measurements are fundamental to measuring VDT display characteristics (for a detailed treatment of photometry and photometric measurements, see Teele, 1965; Smith, 1966; Klein, 1970). The basic unit of photometry is the lumen, which is a measure of visible optical power. To obtain lumen measurements, a photometer is fitted with a filter so that it has the same wavelength sensitivity as the human eye. For the peak of visual sensitivity (at a wavelength of 555 nm), one watt equals 685 lumens. The conversion factor becomes smaller for both longer wavelengths (toward the red) and shorter wavelengths (toward the blue) in accordance with the so-called photopic sensitivity curve.

There are two fundamental photometric parameters for VDTs: luminance and illuminance. All display measurements (with the exception of color) discussed in this section are based on those two parameters. Luminance is the photometric parallel to the sensation of brightness for extended sources; it is a measure of the lumens emitted by a source per solid angle per unit area. The usual CIE (Commission Internationale de l'Eclairage) unit for luminance is the nit (1 candela/m^2) or candela/m^2 (cd/m^2), which this report uses for luminance values (the English unit most commonly used is the foot-Lambert).

Illuminance is a measure of the lumens incident on a surface per unit area. There is no directly parallel visual sensation. The combination of illumination and reflection characteristics of non-light-emitting objects determines the luminance of those objects. The standard CIE unit for illuminance is the lux (1 lumen/m^2), which is the illuminance unit used in this report (the most commonly used English unit is the foot-candle).

Measurement Techniques

Many photometric measuring instruments are commercially available and range from $300 or $400 to more than $10,000. All photometers used to measure luminance have a similar basic construction, consisting of an objective lens, an aperture, a filter, and some type of light-sensing component such as a silicon diode or photomultiplier tube (PMT). The objective lens forms an image of the object being measured at the aperture plane. The aperture is usually a circular hole or a rectangular slit. The light-sensitive element senses only the light that falls on the aperture. The geometry of the instrument is arranged so that the output reading corresponds to the average luminance of the part of the object that is imaged on the aperture. Figure 4.11 shows the arrangement of these components.

Figure 4.12 shows how such a photometer might be mounted and positioned to make measurements on a VDT screen. (It should be noted that normally a photometer such as that shown in Figure 4.12 is located much farther from a VDT when measuring with the lens shown and much closer when measuring with the microscope objective lens.) With the aid of a barium sulfate reflection, the type of photometer shown in Figure 4.12 can also be used to measure illuminance at the VDT screen. Barium sulfate reflects light in a highly diffuse manner and very nearly approximates a perfect diffusing surface. Hence, by positioning the barium sulfate surface at the position at which the illuminance is to be

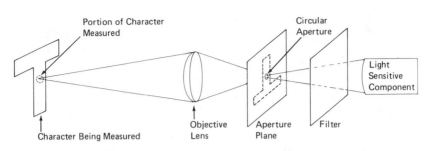

FIGURE 4.11 Components of a typical photometer used for measuring luminance.

measured (as shown in Figure 4.13 for the VDT screen), the luminance of the barium sulfate can be measured and converted to the illuminance at the plane of the material. The illuminance (in lux) can be determined by multiplying the measured luminance in cd/m^2 by the value of π.

We note again that illuminance and luminance are two different types of parameters and one in general cannot be calculated from the other unless the physical and geometric

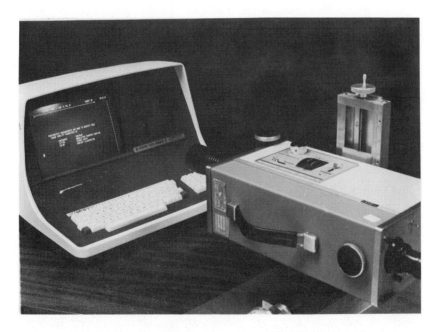

FIGURE 4.12 Photometer mounted to measure VDT screen.

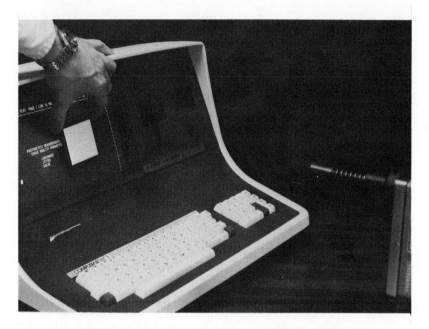

FIGURE 4.13 Measurement of illuminance at the VDT screen.

conditions of the situation are known. In English units, one foot-candle of illumination reflecting from a perfectly white, diffusing reflector gives rise to one foot-Lambert of luminance, and this fact has caused considerable confusion of these two very different parameters.

Measurement of Various Parameters

Character Luminance

The very term character luminance implies that there is a single luminance that is associated with a VDT character. As can be seen in Figure 4.14 the implication is not correct. A character is typically made up of a series of dots and strokes, each of which has a distribution of luminance values across its extent. In general, the linear horizontal strokes (e.g., the top of the letter T and the top, middle, and bottom arms of the letter E) are higher in luminance than the short dots that make up the vertical elements of the characters. While a photometer with microscope objective lens can easily measure any aspect of this luminance distribution, the question is what should be measured and labeled as character

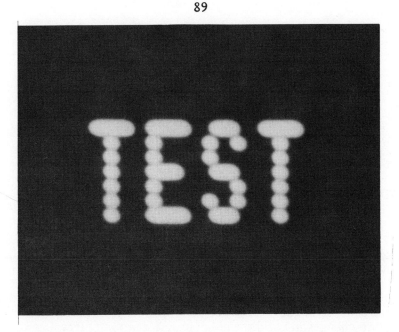

FIGURE 4.14 Light distribution that forms VDT characters.

luminance. There are several options but at present there is no
accepted standard procedure. The three main options include: (1)
a narrow vertical slit (width of the slit much less than the width of
the vertical stroke of character) scan across a vertical character
stroke (such as an I) with the vertical dimension of the slit
covering several dots; (2) the same as above, except that the
vertical height is limited to only one dot or a fraction of one dot;
or (3) a small circular aperture with a diameter much smaller than
the size of a dot. Each measurement will yield a luminance value,
but the most appropriate measurement for determining character
luminance is not apparent.

Character Contrast

To calculate the contrast of a character, it is first necessary to
determine the character luminance and the background luminance. The previous discussion on what constitutes character
luminance obviously applies to the uncertainty associated with
determining contrast. The background luminance is also a problem
because it differs depending on the ambient lighting conditions and
the location on the screen at which the background reading is
made relative to the location of the character or characters. A

TABLE 4.2 Modulation Contrast, Differential Contrast, and Contrast Ratio for Two
Measures of Background Luminance: Hypothetical Case

Measurement Location	Background Luminance (cd/m^2)	Modulation Contrast (%)	Differential Contrast	Contrast Ratio
Far from character	0.5	99	199	200
Near to character	2.0	96	49	50

NOTE: The assumed character luminance is 100 cd/m^2.

CRT screen typically carries a halo of light around characters due
to several light-scattering and stray light sources, which results in
a lower value of measured background luminance the farther from
the character the measurement is made. Dark-room measurements of absolute contrast (calculated by the difference divided
by the sum technique) will not be significantly affected by small
absolute changes in background luminance due to the location of
the measurement. Other values, however, such as differential
contrast (difference divided by background) or the luminance ratio
(also called contrast ratio, or character luminance divided by
background), can change greatly with small changes in absolute
background luminance readings.

To illustrate this effect, Table 4.2 shows a hypothetical set of
data for character luminance and two different background
luminances (one measured near the character and one measured
farther away). Note that the modulation contrast is relatively
insensitive to differences in background luminance compared with
either of the other two calculations for contrast. It is apparent
from the data in Table 4.2 that if a definition of contrast is used
that is highly sensitive to background luminance measurement, the
specific conditions under which background luminance is measured
need to be specified and, preferably, standardized.

Blur, Resolution, and MTF

The terms blur, resolution, and MTF all relate to the definition or
appearance of sharpness of the VDT characters. No accepted
standard procedure exists for measuring these parameters. Whatever procedure is used to measure them, it is still necessary to
select and preferably standardize an appropriate photometer
aperture.

Blur is usually based on a determination of how rapidly the luminance changes with distance at the edge of a character (Dainty and Shaw, 1974; Grandjean and Vigliani, 1980). This is not always easy to determine. Figure 4.15 shows the luminance distribution (measured with a vertical slit and a scanning microphotometer) across a single dot in the character I. It is difficult to define where the edge of either side of the I begins and ends in such a way that repeatable measures can be achieved.

The MTF can be measured in many ways (Schade, 1948; Snyder, 1974; Task and Verona, 1976; Gaskill, 1978). Probably the easiest method for VDT screens is by using the edge-response or line-response techniques described in Gaskill (1978). These methods are preferred because no special, separate signal generation devices are required; instead, selected VDT characters can serve as the input signals. For example, if the input signal is the narrowest vertical line that the VDT is capable of producing, then the luminance profile shown in Figure 4.15 is the line spread function (LSF) for the VDT. The MTF of the VDT can then be calculated by taking the normalized Fourier transform of the LSF, as described in Gaskill (1978).

An alternative technique is to measure the edge response of some selected character on a VDT. This technique does not

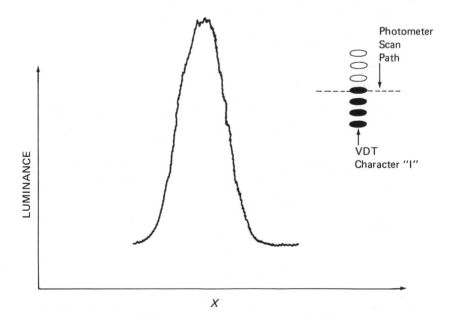

FIGURE 4.15 Luminance distribution across a single dot in the character I.

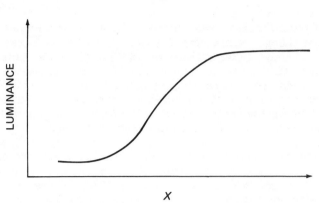

FIGURE 4.16 Typical edge response (luminance distribution at the edge of a character).

require the assumption that the selected character represents the narrowest line possible, as does the LSF technique. It does, however, require an additional mathematical step. The edge response is simply the luminance distribution measured at the edge of a character. A typical edge response may look like that shown in Figure 4.16. The curve is first differentiated, which yields the line spread function, and then the normalized Fourier transform is taken to obtain the MTF (as described above).

Reflection Characteristics

As described in the section "Filters for VDTs," there are two types of reflections that occur with VDTs: specular and diffuse. Specular reflection occurs from the front surface of the screen and satisfies the optical law that the angle of incidence of a light ray on a surface equals the angle of reflection. Diffuse reflection is a scattering in all directions of the incident light and occurs at the phosphor surface of the VDT. There are no accepted, standardized procedures to measure either of these parameters.

The specular reflection coefficients for the data presented in Tables 4.1, 4.5, and 4.6 were obtained using the following procedure. A light box, measuring approximately 20 x 25 cm, was positioned 1.5 m from a VDT screen and tilted at an angle of about 17° from a straight line from the center of the VDT screen (see Figure 4.17). The photometer was located about 17° on the other side of the straight-line position and focused on the VDT screen. The luminance of the reflection was measured and divided by the luminance of the light box. It should be noted that much of the light from the light box was transmitted through the front surface of the VDT screen and fell on the diffuse phosphor surface. The measurement was not, therefore, a pure specular reflectance coefficient because of the diffusely scattered light in the area measured. It is extremely difficult to avoid this situation entirely. Since the effect depends on the size of the light box used and its distance from the VDT, it is necessary to specify these parameters in order to make meaningful comparisons between VDTs.

Determining the diffuse reflection coefficient is somewhat more involved. The phosphor surface acts as a fairly good diffusing surface, but it is by no means a perfect diffuser. Consequently, the amount of light diffusely reflected depends both on the angle of the photometer with respect to the VDT surface and the angle of the light source with respect to the VDT surface. A geometry should be chosen that is representative of the viewing and illumination conditions typically encountered in VDT use. For the measurements shown in Tables 4.5 and 4.6, the photometer was located directly in front of the VDT screen, simulating an operator's view. The illuminating light source consisted of overhead room lights and a slide projector located about 45° from the straight-line position (see Figure 4.18). The resulting illumination at the VDT screen was approximately 400 lux, near the mid-range of the 300-500 lux recommended for office work areas. The illumination was measured using the barium sulfate technique described in the section "Measurement Techniques." The diffuse reflectance coefficient was calculated by dividing the resulting screen luminance (using a blank screen) by the incident illumination.

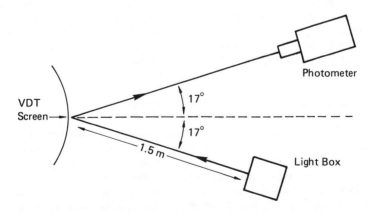

FIGURE 4.17 Geometry for measuring specular reflection.

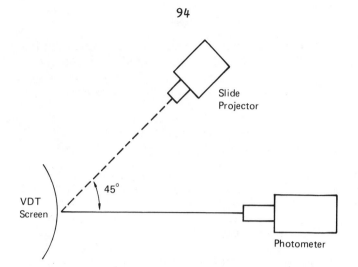

FIGURE 4.18 Geometry used for measuring diffuse reflectance coefficient.

Since individual characters are not measured in determining the reflection characteristics, the choice of photometer aperture is not critical.

Standardization

As is apparent from the preceding discussion, there are currently no standard procedures for measuring the critical display quality characteristics of VDTs. Standard procedures should be developed so that accurate comparisons of image quality among VDTs can be made. Once this is accomplished, recommended values for these parameters should be established to provide guidelines for determining the image quality of any particular VDT.

FLAT-PANEL DISPLAYS

Most of the concern about VDTs centers on the cathode-ray tube, currently the most common display device in VDTs. However, a growing proportion of terminals replace the CRT with a flat-panel, solid-state display device. While analysis of the engineering details and advantages of flat-panel displays is beyond the purposes of this report, it should be recognized that these devices may have distinct advantages over the CRT. Flat-panel displays take up less display depth and can therefore be located more conveniently on a display surface of limited size. In addition, since each picture element (pixel) on a flat-panel display is defined by the location of electrodes or similar elements, the picture is geometrically stable and does not move from frame to frame or over time. The following section describes the main variables related to visual perception of the dot-matrix display structure used in flat-panel displays and indicates what is known about the relationship between these variables and visual task performance. Since the basic physiological effects of the various display variables (luminance, contrast, flicker, etc.) are the same for flat-panel displays as for CRTs, this section is limited to a discussion of the relationships between display design variables and performance.

Dot-Matrix Display Variables

Character Size Effects

In general, the size of the display should be adequate to present the necessary information for the task required of the operator. There are no standard requirements for screen size, but there are requirements for sizes of the information elements presented on the screen. Thus, as the task requires a greater amount of information, the screen generally increases in size to accommodate the larger amount of information, each element of which must be presented at a suitable size.

It has been shown that the proper character size varies with the nature of the task. For example, visual search for individual characters is improved as the size of the character gets larger. Snyder and Maddox (1978) showed that increases in individual dot sizes up to 1.50 mm improved random search time (Figure 4.19). They also showed that a dot size of 1.50 mm is greater than optimum for continuous reading of text (Figure 4.20). In essence, if the characters are too large, reading time is reduced because of the increase in necessary eye movements and numbers of visual fixations. On the other hand, larger characters are desirable in a search-type display, simply because peripheral characters can apparently be more easily located in peripheral vision. A meaningful standard at the present time appears to be that offered by the proposed German TCA specification, which requires a minimum character size of 2.6 mm or 18 min of arc, whichever is greater.

There is a large variability among observers and among tasks in viewing distance, and the character size must be compatible with the viewing distance. The above specification takes this into account. It generally assumes that the minimum viewing distance

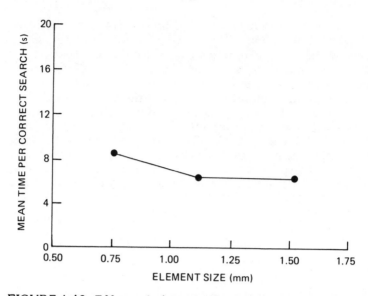

FIGURE 4.19 Effect of element size on random search time. SOURCE: Snyder and Maddox (1978).

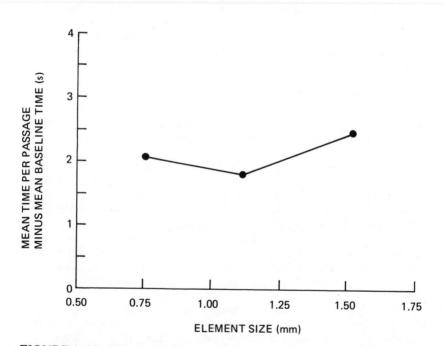

FIGURE 4.20 Effect of element size on reading time. SOURCE: Snyder and Maddox (1978).

will be 50 cm, although longer viewing distances are feasible for some particular tasks and workplace geometries. If a longer viewing distance can be anticipated, then the greater character size necessary to meet the 18 minutes of arc requirement is justified.

Character sizes should not be obtained at the cost of a reduction in image quality (see below). For example, it can be demonstrated that increasing the character size by increasing the pitch of the raster lines in a CRT display is detrimental because the visibility of raster lines significantly reduces performance even though the character size is increased.

Character Formation

In general, as for CRT displays, stroke-written characters are preferred to characters having visible dot or element structure (see discussion in the section "Raster Structure").

Where dot-matrix characters are used, there are known trade-offs among the design characteristics of the characters. In particular, the dot size and shape interact in a unique fashion. In all cases, vertical elongation of dots should be avoided; dots approaching a square aspect ratio are most desirable. This has been shown in several experiments, such as that summarized in Figure 4.21. When the shape of the dot is combined with what is known regarding spacing between elements (see discussion in the section "Raster Structure"), it is apparent that the best display design has square dots that are essentially adjacent to one another.

The size of the dot matrix or the number of video lines in a raster display used to form the individual characters is equally important. Figure 4.22 shows that the optimum matrix size depends on the character font used. As discussed above, a 7 x 9 character is generally more legible than a 5 x 7 character and a 9 x 11 character is more legible than a 7 x 9 one. Also, the more dots or elements available to form the character the better the individual legibility of the character, although diminishing returns appear to be reached beyond matrix sizes of 9 x 11. Similar results have been obtained with raster scan displays.

In recent years, there has been some interest in describing the intermittency of characters using a measure called percent active area, which is simply the proportion of the total display space which is illuminated by the dots. The percent active area is the square of the ratio of the dot diameter to the center-to-center dot spacing, multiplied by 100. As shown in Figure 4.23, increases in the percent active area lead to reductions in character recognition error rates. Under adverse reading conditions, active areas in excess of 50 percent are desirable, while under normal conditions

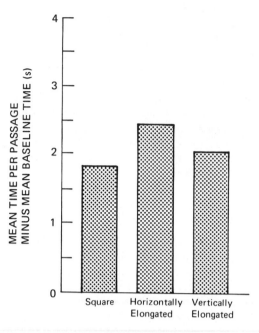

ELEMENT SHAPE

FIGURE 4.21 Effect of element shape on reading time. SOURCE: Snyder and Maddox (1978).

active areas in excess of 30 percent appear to achieve asymptotic performance. In general, the percent active area measure is not critical if good design practice is followed by reducing space between character dots.

Contrast

Maximum legibility can be achieved for contextual (e.g., text) displays when the modulation is at least 75 percent.[3] Very little gain is achieved beyond 75 percent. If the information presented on the display is noncontextual (e.g., isolated numerals or letters),

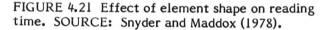

[3]Modulation, one of several quantitative measures of contrast, is equal to the difference between character and background luminance divided by the sum of the two.

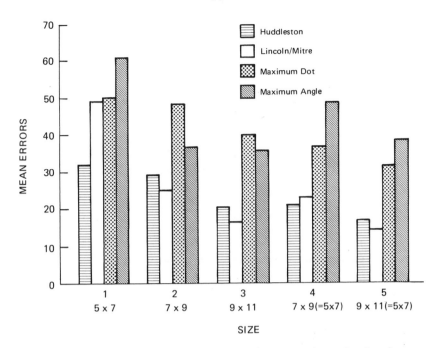

FIGURE 4.22 Interaction of font and character/matrix size in determining single character legibility. SOURCE: Snyder and Maddox (1978).

a modulation of at least 90 percent is required to avoid reductions in legibility. It should be noted that these values of modulation are referenced to the display as viewed by the operator and therefore take into account the ambient illuminance and any reflections. Glare reduction, good workplace illumination design, and high intrinsic contrast of the display are all necessary to achieve an acceptable contrast level.

Characters with sharper edges, or less blur, are generally more legible than those with greater blur or reduced sharpness. Unfortunately, adequate measures of sharpness and their relationship to legibility are not well established. It has been shown that reductions in object identification occur when the blur exceeds one-half of the width of the individual item, but these data apply to various cultural objects rather than to alphanumeric characters. Studies should be performed in which text reading and legibility, rather than object recognition, are the primary tasks.

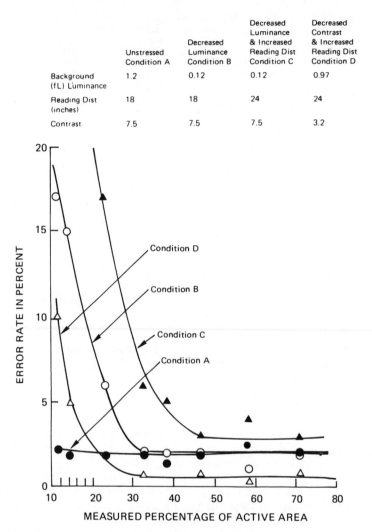

	Unstressed Condition A	Decreased Luminance Condition B	Decreased Luminance & Increased Reading Dist Condition C	Decreased Contrast & Increased Reading Dist Condition D
Background (fL) Luminance	1.2	0.12	0.12	0.97
Reading Dist (inches)	18	18	24	24
Contrast	7.5	7.5	7.5	3.2

FIGURE 4.23 Effect of percent active area on character recognition. SOURCE: Stein (1980).

Font

The legibility of displayed alphanumeric information is greatly dependent on the character style or font. Legibility also interacts with the size of the matrix and the overall character size. As illustrated in Figure 4.22, the Huddleston font is the most legible of those studied for 5 x 7 characters, but the Huddleston and

Lincoln/Mitre fonts are equally legible for either 7 x 9 or 9 x 11 matrix sizes. Since there is absolutely no standardization of fonts across existing systems, care should be taken by designers and users to select fonts that give optimum legibility rather than unique character designs. Generalizations from existing literature pertaining to stroke-written characters (e.g., printed text) appear reasonable and should be followed until more directly related data are generated.

Luminance Uniformity

Uniformity considerations are similar to those discussed previously in this chapter for CRT displays.

Information Density

Research relating the minimum, maximum, and optimum densities of information in the vertical and horizontal dimensions is urgently needed. Currently, word processing and data processing displays range from a few lines through a more typical 24 lines per display height to a full page of approximately 60 lines. The displays vary in physical size, and the characters also vary in size. It is clear that full-page displays are desirable for formatting purposes, but they are often very difficult to read because of the resulting small character size. Similarly, it is obvious that large character sizes on partial page displays produce legible characters but that formatting is a difficult and often tiring task. There are no useful guidelines from the literature to suggest optimum levels of display information density, and we strongly recommend research in this area.

Dot-Matrix Display Quality Measures

While image quality measures have been researched in some depth for CRT displays, very little attention has been given to suitable measures of image quality for flat-panel displays. Although it may at first seem reasonable to assume that such measures should be approximately the same, the very nature of the differences between the two displays suggests that the metrics designed to accommodate continuous information, as is the case with the CRT, cannot often be used to describe information that is presented discretely. This section summarizes briefly the only research done to date that has attempted to summarize image quality for dot-matrix displays.

TABLE 4.3   Pool of Predictor Variables

Vertical	Horizontal	Description
VFREQ	HFREQ	Fundamental spatial frequency (cyc/deg)
VFLOG	HFLOG	Base 10 log of fundamental spatial frequency
VSQR	HSQR	Square of (fundamental spatial frequency minus 14.0)
VMOD	HMOD	Modulation of fundamental spatial frequency
VDIV	HDIV	Fundamental spatial frequency divided by modulation
VLOG	HLOG	Base 10 log of VDIV and HDIV
VMTFA	HMTFA	Pseudo-modulation-transfer-function area
VMLOG	HMLOG	Base 10 log of VMTFA and HMTFA
MCROS	HCROS	Spatial frequency at which modulation curve crosses the threshold curve
VRANG	HRANG	Crossover frequency minus fundamental frequency

SOURCE: Snyder and Maddox (1978).

In a three-year research program, Snyder and Maddox (1978) summarized the best possible prediction of image quality and visual task performance from a variety of geometric and photometric variables that were measured from flat-panel displays. The pool of predictor variables is shown in Table 4.3. These variables were all measured physically from a variety of flat-panel displays from which human visual task performance data were collected. The data pertained to two visual tasks, a reading task and a visual search task for randomly appearing alphanumerics. The predictor variables shown in Table 4.3 were then entered into a linear stepwise multiple regression equation, to obtain the best prediction equation for both the reading and the visual search tasks. The resulting prediction equations are shown in Table 4.4. From this table it can be seen that the prediction equation predicts reading time to an accuracy of approximately 53 percent of the total variance among display types, and the equation for search time predicts approximately 50 percent of the variability among different displays. It would appear that these predictability proportions can be improved with further research, but it is also clear that it is necessary to make careful and detailed measurements of displays to achieve this level of predictability. Further research is clearly indicated to obtain a greater understanding of the relationship between visual task performance and the design of flat-panel displays.

TABLE 4.4   Extended Predictive Equations

Task	Metric and Related Information
Reading Time	Adjusted Reading Time (s) = 5.74 + 0.3111(HFREQ) + 2.479(HMOD) + 4.365(HLOG) − 14.973(HFLOG) + 1.112(VMLOG) Correlation Coefficient R = .72 $R^2 = .525$ Asymptotic $R^2 = .637$
Search Time	Search Time (s) = 7.27 + 0.027(HDIV) + 2.159(HLOG) + 5.916(VFLOG) − 0.339(VMTFA) − 0.054(VRANG) + 5.487(VMLOG) Correlation Coefficient R = .71 $R^2 = .500$ Asymptotic $R^2 = .575$

SOURCE: Snyder and Maddox (1978).

Advantages and Disadvantages of Flat-Panel Displays Compared With CRTs

A flat-panel display is usually only 1 to 2 in. deep, while the CRT used in most terminals is on the order of 12 to 18 in. deep. Thus, for a given desk size, a flat-panel display can be located farther from an operator than a CRT display and may therefore be helpful in preventing problems with accommodation. The flat-panel display is also usually lighter weight and can therefore be moved more readily.

A flat-panel display has a fixed image location, which does not vary with voltage irregularities, and it does not have deflection circuit inadequacies and some of the other ills that plague CRT displays. It has been suggested by some that the better image stability of flat displays may help significantly reduce ocular discomfort reported by users of CRT VDTs; however, there has been no research directly addressing this suggestion. Greater contrast can be obtained on some flat-panel displays in comparison with CRTs. This is often desirable in an environment that has high ambient illumination.

The major disadvantage of a flat-panel display is its extremely high cost relative to a CRT. At the present time, the few flat-panel displays that would meet the requirements of current data processing and word processing terminals cost in excess of $3,000--prohibitive compared with the cost of typical CRT displays. Thus, it may be some time before widespread use of flat-panel displays is seen in the VDT environment.

FILTERS FOR VDTs

The contrast-reducing effects of reflections can be partially
controlled by the use of various optical and physical techniques. If
these techniques are not used and if the ambient lighting
conditions cannot be properly controlled, it may be advisable to
use a filter over the screen. Many types of filters are available,
ranging from less than $5 to more than $100 and having an equal
range of effectiveness. The purpose of these filters is to improve
the legibility of the display by improving the contrast or reducing
glare: in most cases "glare" refers to specular reflections from
the front surface of the VDT. Both diffuse and specular reflections from VDT screens were discussed in the section "Reflection
Characteristics." This section describes several types of filters
that are currently available and discusses their effectiveness.

Kinds of Filters

Circular Polarizer with Antireflection Coating

A circular polarizer filter with antireflection coating can be used
to reduce both specular and diffuse reflections. It is the most
expensive filter available and probably one of the most effective.

The outside surface of this type of filter is coated with several
layers of optically transparent materials to form what is called an
antireflection coating. The effect of the coating is to significantly reduce specular reflections from the surface of the filter.
The rest of the filter package consists of substrate material
(typically glass) sandwiched around the more delicate components,
a linear polarizer and a quarter-wave plate. The linear polarizer
and the quarter-wave plate together form what is commonly
known as a circular polarizer. The circular polarizer converts
unpolarized incident light to circularly polarized light. The light
is changed from right-handed circularly polarized light to left-
handed circularly polarized light (or vice versa) on reflection from
the VDT screen. Because of the optical physics of the circular
polarizer, the light is blocked from getting back through the filter
in much the same way that light is blocked by crossed linear
polarizers.

This type of filter reduces specular reflections in two ways: by
reducing specular reflections from the filter itself through the use
of the antireflection coating and by eliminating specular
reflections from the underlying VDT screen through use of the
circular polarizer. Diffuse reflections are reduced primarily by
the light attenuation effects of the polarizer material, which
allows only about 35 percent of the incident unpolarized light to

pass through the filter to the phosphor surface of the VDT screen. The light is diffusely scattered by the phosphor surface, thus losing most of its polarization characteristics; and it is again reduced to about 35 percent as it passes back through the filter toward the user. This process results in an improvement of the display contrast since the ambient incident light (illumination) is attenuated twice by the filter (once as it arrives at the screen and again as it diffusely reflects through the filter toward the operator), while the VDT character luminance is attenuated only once as it passes through the filter to the operator.

Neutral Density Filters

A neutral density filter is probably the simplest of the contrast enhancement filters. It typically consists of a neutrally tinted plastic that allows the passage of some percentage (usually 15-25 percent) of the light that falls on it. This filter is most effective in reducing diffuse reflections. Light from ambient sources is attenuated twice as it passes through the filter to the VDT phosphor surface and is reflected from the phosphor surface through the filter toward the operator. Since the light from the VDT characters passes through the filter only once, the display contrast is improved.

Specular reflections may not be reduced by this type of filter unless the surface of the filter is treated with an antireflection coating (as discussed above) or with a matte finish coating that blurs the specular reflections.

A filter that is apparently not commonly available but that would appear to be both effective and inexpensive is a neutral density filter formed into a spherical concave shape. Because such a shape is opposite in direction to the curvature of the VDT screen, the edges of the filter would have to be located a short distance from the screen. If the radius of curvature of the screen were approximately equal to the operator's viewing distance, and the screen were tilted somewhat below the operator's eye level, reflection sources would be limited to the operator's chest and abdominal areas. And if those areas were kept somewhat dark, for example by an operator's wearing dark clothing, specular reflections should not be a problem. Diffuse reflections would be reduced as they are with any neutral density filter.

A filter based on the physical curvature of the filter material is described in U.S. Patent 3,744,893 entitled "Viewing Device with Filter Means for Optimizing Image Quality" issued to Chandler (1973). As described, the filter was intended for use with a film viewing device but could be adapted to VDTs.

Notch or Color Filters

Notch or color filters are designed to allow transmission of a high percentage of incident light of some specified wavelengths (typically in the green portion of the spectrum) and a high absorption at other wavelengths. The principle of this type of filter is essentially the same as that of a neutral density filter, but in notch or color filters the bandpass (color) is tuned to the VDT screen color. A green filter placed over a VDT with a green phosphor will allow most of the display luminance to pass through the filter to the operator, while ambient illumination, which is usually broadband white, is largely absorbed by the filter (except for the green portion). This process reduces the ambient light that causes diffuse reflections on the VDT screen, thus improving contrast.

As is the case with neutral density filters, control of specular reflections with this type of filter depends on the surface treatment of the filter.

Directional Filters

Directional filters use geometric or optical means to prevent ambient light from reaching the VDT or to prevent reflections from reaching the user. One type of directional filter is composed of a thin sheet of material with tiny, opaque, imbedded slats that are perpendicular to the surface of the sheet. The slats act as a miniature venetian blind, allowing light to travel only in certain directions. When the slats are oriented toward the operator, light from the VDT can pass to the operator but light from overhead cannot reach the VDT screen. This process reduces contrast loss due to diffuse reflections. Specular reflections would have to be reduced by surface treatment of the filter, as described above.

Evaluation of Filters

General Comments

Some general characteristics of filters should be noted. First, antireflection coatings tend to be somewhat delicate and will typically degrade with time, use, and cleaning. Second, plastics used in filters are softer than glass, and they also become scratched and degrade with time, thus reducing the effectiveness of the filter.

TABLE 4.5   Effect of Several Filters on Contrast and Luminance of VDT Characters for a Smooth-Finish VDT Screen

Filter	Dark Room		Specular Reflection[a]		Diffuse Reflection[b]	
	Contrast (%)	Luminance (cd/m^2)	Contrast (%)	Luminance (cd/m^2)	Contrast (%)	Luminance (cd/m^2)
None	98.8	115.0	26.1	330.0	66.4	178.0
1	97.6	28.7	17.4	115.0	65.9	45.8
2	98.1	36.3	24.5	116.0	67.1	56.4
3	96.9	21.9	16.6	92.7	69.2	32.8
4	98.3	41.3	21.1	139.0	70.9	58.1
5	98.2	36.9	28.9	99.2	81.6	50.6
6	99.2	41.7	34.9	95.8	81.3	58.1
7	99.0	34.2	11.8	195.0	80.6	47.9

[a] Illumination at screen, 266 lux; luminance of specular reflection source, 2,950 cd/m^2
[b] Illumination at screen, 413 lux; luminance of specular reflection source, none.

Third, matte-surface treatments are not very effective in dealing with specular reflections in terms of their effect on contrast, although they do reduce the sharpness of specular reflections. Unfortunately, matte finishes reduce the sharpness of the display characters as well, and this effect increases the farther from the VDT surface the filter is located. Some loss in character sharpness may be helpful, however, in reducing the dot structure of characters (see data on filters 1, 2, 3, and 4 in Tables 4.5 and 4.6).

Fourth, VDT screens are convex, curved surfaces and are therefore susceptible to specular reflections that are visible to the operator over a very wide range of angles (see Figure 4.24a). If a flat or concave filter is placed over the screen, the angles over which specular reflections may occur are drastically reduced and therefore more easily controlled (see Figure 4.24b), a subtle but signficant advantage for such filters.

Effectiveness of Filters

Because the effectiveness of a particular filter depends on many variables and combinations of variables, it is not possible to fully discuss the issue of effectivensss in this report. For a limited comparison of the effectiveness of several filters and filter types, we measured the effects of seven filters on two different types of CRT screens:

TABLE 4.6 Effect of Several Filters on Contrast and Luminance of VDT Characters for a Matte-Finish VDT Screen

Filter	Dark Room Contrast (%)	Luminance (cd/m²)	Specular Reflection[a] Plus Room Lights Contrast (%)	Luminance (cd/m²)	Diffuse Reflection[b] Plus Room Lights Contrast (%)	Luminance (cd/m²)
None	99.5	130.0	35.2	248.0	78.9	145.0
1	98.0	33.5	17.5	110.0	71.0	38.3
2	98.4	43.1	24.0	107.0	77.6	48.7
3	97.4	25.6	16.1	94.7	78.7	28.7
4	98.5	46.2	23.4	128.0	81.7	51.0
5	98.4	43.1	30.7	90.3	85.5	43.8
6	98.6	46.9	36.5	88.9	87.0	49.2
7	98.2	37.3	11.3	185.0	83.1	40.7

[a] Illumination at screen, 293 lux; luminance of specular reflection source, 2,950 cd/m²
[b] illumination at screen, 428 lux; luminance of specular reflection source, none.

1. Amber filter with matte finish (curved)
2. Gray filter with matte finish (curved)
3. Green filter with matte finish (curved)
4. Neutral filter with matte finish (curved)
5. Circular polarizer with antireflection coating (flat)--manufacturer A
6. Circular polarizer with antireflection coating (flat)--manufacturer B
7. Green filter with smooth finish (flat)

The filters were measured under three conditions: in total darkness, in the presence of a specular source, and in the presence of a diffuse reflection source. The specular reflection source was a light box with a luminance of approximately 2,950 cd/m² positioned approximately 1.5 m from the VDT screen and approximately 17° off-axis (see Figure 4.25). Measurements under the specular reflection condition were taken with the room lights on, thus this condition was not one of a pure specular reflection. The diffuse reflection condition was achieved with a combination of normal room lights and a slide projector located off to one side to provide nonspecularly reflecting illumination (specular and diffuse reflections on a typical VDT screen are shown in Figure 4.10). The illumination at the plane of the screen (which results in loss of contrast due to diffuse reflection) was measured under each of the three conditions. The measurements are shown in Tables 4.5 and 4.6.

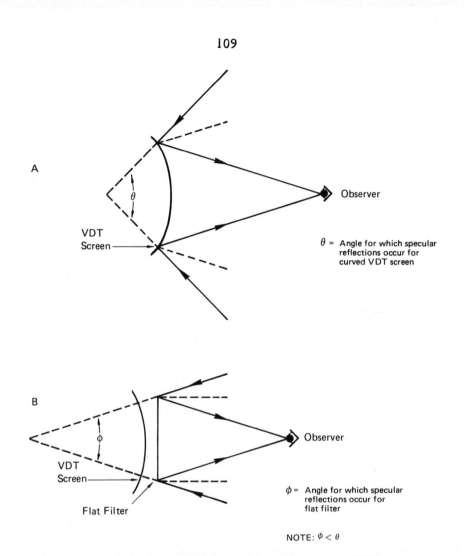

A

Observer

θ = Angle for which specular
reflections occur for
curved VDT screen

VDT
Screen

B

Observer

ϕ = Angle for which specular
reflections occur for
flat filter

VDT
Screen

Flat Filter

NOTE: $\phi < \theta$

FIGURE 4.24 Specular reflection angles for a curved VDT screen (a) and for a flat VDT filter (b).

The contrast and the luminance of the VDT characters were measured without a filter on two different types of VDT screens. Table 4.5 shows the measurements made on a VDT screen with a smooth surface; Table 4.6 shows the measurements on a screen with a matte surface.

There are several items worthy of special note in the data of Tables 4.5 and 4.6. Displays with both smooth and matte finishes have extremely high contrast in a dark room; it is the ambient

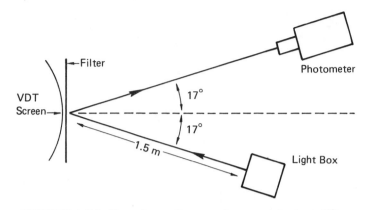

FIGURE 4.25 Top view of geometry used to test filter effectiveness against specular reflections.

environmental lighting that causes a loss of contrast. All filters reduce the luminance of the display characters. This means that when a filter is used, the VDT must be operated at a higher beam current to achieve the same character luminance as when no filter is used. The increased beam current causes the phosphor to age (become less efficient) more rapidly and reduces the lifetime of a CRT.

For the smooth-finish screen (Table 4.5), the circular polarizer filters improved contrast under the specular reflection condition; the improvement, however, was only moderate. For the matte-finish screen (Table 4.6), under the specular reflection condition, none of the filters resulted in a significant improvement over the no-filter condition. For both the smooth-finish and matte-finish screens, several filters improved the contrast under the diffuse reflection condition compared with the no-filter condition, but again the improvement was only moderate.

Filters 1, 2, and 3 not only did not improve contrast for either the smooth-finish or matte-finish screens, but resulted in poorer contrast under several conditions. Since the phosphor used in both VDTs was a P-4 white phosphor, these results indicate that color filters might not be expected to improve contrast unless the filter color is matched to that of the phosphor. Filter 7 (green, flat, smooth finish), however, performed well under the diffuse reflection condition, but very poorly under the specular reflection condition. In general, filters are more effective in reducing diffuse reflections than in reducing specular reflections. This is unfortunate because specular reflections cause the greater loss of contrast and probably contribute more to problems encountered in viewing VDTs.

5
Lighting and Reflections

Experience reveals that lighting and reflections may cause problems for video display terminal operators. The reflection of a lamp or a bright window on any viewing screen makes it difficult or impossible to see the picture. Even if the picture is visible through the glare, the reflection may be distracting and annoying. Almost everyone who has watched television or worked at a VDT, microfilm viewer, or similar display device has probably had such experiences. Many complaints reported by VDT operators are specifically related to workplace lighting and reflections. Several studies involving such complaints are reviewed and analyzed later in this chapter.

The basic principles and most of the details of how lighting and reflections affect visual performance and comfort are known. Lighting specification systems based on principles of geometry, the physics of light and reflectance, and characteristics of the human visual system are routinely used by illuminating engineers and other lighting specialists to design appropriate lighting for workplaces. Good lighting design also includes esthetic and other considerations intended to promote appropriate psychological and social reactions. Although lighting specification systems differ in their specific assumptions, criteria, and spatial resolution, they are fundamentally the same. An experienced, well-trained lighting specialist could use these systems to design appropriate lighting for VDT workplaces and to predict or explain problems that may result from inappropriate lighting design.

Workplaces in which VDTs are used require lighting designs that differ in simple ways from those required in non-VDT workplaces. The differences primarily involve geometrical relationships--the presence of VDTs may complicate lighting design by adding (or substituting) work surfaces in different positions and planes.

111

Just as some workplaces are poorly designed in terms of lighting and workstation arrangements for non-VDT work, so some are poorly designed for VDT work. It is likely that many offices designed for desk-top paperwork are now being used for VDT work without appropriate modifications of the lighting. Higher rates of complaints for work involving VDTs compared to other types of work may largely be due to inappropriate lighting for the VDT situations. As lighting is improved for VDT installations, many of the problems attributed to VDTs may vanish.

ILLUMINATION

Illumination in offices and other workplaces comes from light sources, windows, and reflections from a variety of objects and surfaces. VDTs differ from most other task objects or surfaces in that they emit light, and they usually have a highly specular curved glass surface in a more vertical plane. These differences have important consequences with respect to illumination and reflections. For example, VDT operators in some situations see reflections of their faces and clothing on the display screen. Such reflections can be annoying and distracting, and in some cases may reduce task visibility enough to affect performance. An analysis of the basic characteristics of illumination should be helpful in determining the possible role each may play in causing problems for VDT operators.

The four major characteristics of illumination are spectral composition, temporal changes, intensity, and spatial or directional aspects. There is little indication or reason to believe that spectral composition or temporal changes of illumination are responsible for complaints or problems peculiar to VDT use. Illumination having unusual or extreme color or flicker characteristics may interact with display characteristics in special ways that may cause problems. (Display characteristics, including color and flicker, are discussed in Chapter 4.) It is unlikely that such conditions were involved in any of the studies reviewed in this report. Although some people have negative attitudes and reactions to commonly used illumination (certain spectral compositions and flicker frequencies), there is no indication that these conditions have special importance in VDT situations.

For the other two major characteristics of illumination, intensity and spatial aspects, there are important differences between VDT and non-VDT work situations. Our review and analysis of these characteristics of illumination is divided into three parts: problems caused by successive viewing of different luminances (which can lead to transient adaptation), reflections, and glare.

Transient Adaptation

Transient adaptation refers to the temporary loss in visibility that occurs when a person changes his or her point of regard to surfaces having different luminances or when illumination changes occur naturally in the visual environment. In general, the greater the ratio of change or difference in luminance levels, the greater the loss in visibility (Boynton et al., 1969; Rinalducci and Beare, 1974, 1975).

The results of research on transient adaptation have typically been interpreted in terms of the ratio of the contrast threshold of the target in the transient state of adaptation to the contrast threshold after complete adaptation to the new prevailing luminance level. This ratio (symbolized by ϕ) represents the increased amount of light needed to see the target in the transient versus the steady state and thus is indicative of loss in visibility as a function of luminance change. Figure 5.1 shows ϕ as a function of the ratio of background field change. Figure 5.2 shows log ϕ and ϕ plotted as a function of the log ratio of background field change and compares data obtained by Boynton and coworkers (1969) and Rinalducci and Beare (1974). Here, as with most research of this nature, the transient state threshold is measured 300 msec (τ) after the change from the prevailing luminance level, B_1, to the new luminance level, B_2.

Visibility losses due to transient adaptation in VDT operations occur when an operator looks toward a glare source (e.g., a window or a luminaire) and then back to the display screen. The decrement in visibility should be particularly large for a positive-contrast display (light characters on a dark background). A second situation that could involve losses in visibility due to transient adaptation is when a positive-contrast display is combined with a negative-contrast source document, such as a typewritten page. Visibility losses may also occur when secondary task lighting is used on the source document. In this situation, a VDT operator using a positive-contrast display may be particularly prone to the effects of transient adaptation, especially when a negative-contrast source document is used. Rupp (1981) has reviewed a number of European and Canadian documents that recommend standards for VDT design and use. Two of the documents reviewed--a report of the Technical University of Berlin (Cakir et al., 1978) and the German DIN draft Standard 66234--express some concern with transient adaptation effects that may occur when an operator continually looks back and forth between a positive-contrast display and a negative-contrast source document. Rupp appears unconvinced that such effects are significant, citing the review of MacLeod (1978) and the research on scotopic adaptation

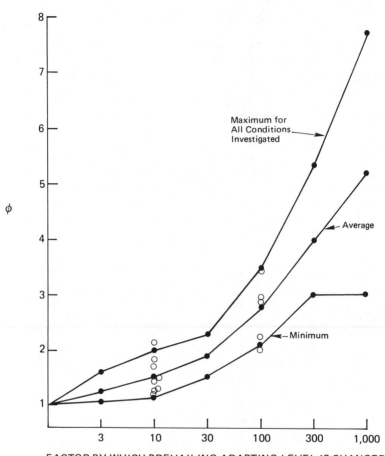

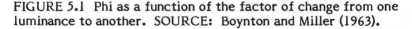

FACTOR BY WHICH PREVAILING ADAPTING LEVEL IS CHANGED

FIGURE 5.1 Phi as a function of the factor of change from one luminance to another. SOURCE: Boynton and Miller (1963).

by Barlow and Andrews (1973), and suggests that the visual system's level of adaptation is determined by the luminance of the light symbols and not by an integrated luminance level or background luminance level. Thus, if this hypothesis is correct, one might be more concerned with matching the luminance of the light symbols with the source document background. However, the evidence presented in support of Rupp's hypothesis is either unconvincing or inappropriate, and we believe the situation needs to be examined further (also see the discussion in Chapter 4).

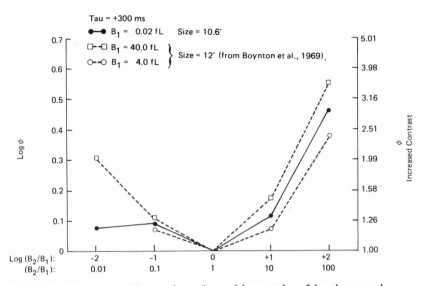

FIGURE 5.2   Log phi as a function of log ratio of backgrounds.
Data from an experiment employing the same ratios by Boynton et
al. (1969) are included to allow comparison with effects of similar
changes from higher initial luminances. NOTE: The right-hand
ordinate and lower abscissa scales make the figure direct-reading
for phi as a function of the ratio of the backgrounds. SOURCE:
Rinalducci and Beare (1974).

Reflections

CRT screens are usually convex, spherical shells of glass with a
radius of curvature of approximately 63.5 cm. Reflections from
the mirrorlike front surface of the screen form images. A very
distant object seen by reflection in the screen will appear to be
located at one-half the distance from the screen to its center of
curvature, i.e., at 31.75 cm behind the screen. For an operator at
70 cm from the screen, dioptric accommodation levels for the
screen and the reflected image are 1.43 diopters and 0.98 diopter,
respectively. The reflected image of an object located close to
the screen will also be closer to the plane of the CRT face. For
example, if an operator at 70 cm from the screen sees his or her
face reflected from the screen, the image will appear to be
located about 22 cm behind the screen. Reflected images of
luminaires or windows can produce a veil of light (reflected glare)
over a portion of the screen. They can also serve as distracting or
annoying stimuli that may cause discomfort or affect performance indirectly by distracting or changing the motivation of the

operator (see Petherbridge and Hopkinson, 1955, for evidence from a non-VDT study).

Since reflected images form at distances other than that of the screen surface, accommodation and convergence may fluctuate or otherwise be inappropriate for viewing the screen. This effect may be annoying, induce discomfort, or affect performance. Reflected images may also affect performance if an operator looks directly at them (possibly due to phototropism), which could cause transient adaptation problems (DeBoer, 1977). Reflected images could also induce binocular rivalry, which might cause discomfort or affect task performance (Reitmaier, 1979).

The inside phosphor surface of a CRT screen reflects light in a diffuse manner rather than imaging it. Light also excites the phosphor, increasing its illuminance. Both effects can reduce contrast. Many VDTs have adjustments for screen brightness (illuminance) and contrast that can compensate for this type of effect except in extreme cases.

An analysis and discussion of relationships between problems reported by VDT operators, such as ocular discomfort and fatigue, and physiological optics variables, such as accommodation, fixation, convergence, and binocular rivalry, is included in Chapter 7.

Glare

Glare is the sensation produced by luminances within the visual field that are sufficiently greater than the luminance to which the eyes are adapted to cause annoyance, discomfort, or loss in visual performance and visibility (Kaufman and Christensen, 1972). The magnitude of the sensation of glare depends on factors such as the size, position, and luminance of the light source or reflecting surface, the number of light sources, and the luminance to which the eyes are adapted. Reflected glare is the result of specular reflections from polished or glossy surfaces or diffuse reflections that produce a veil of light that reduces contrast. Disability glare, which may be caused by light scattered within the eye (reducing contrast at the retina), or by reflected glare, reduces visual performance and visibility. Discomfort glare produces discomfort, and it may, but does not necessarily, interfere with visual performance or visibility, just as disability glare may or may not be accompanied by discomfort.

The large reported differences among individuals in sensitivity to glare, as well as the great variability among studies, may be due to problems in methodology, especially in studies of discomfort glare (see, e.g., Lulla and Bennett, 1981). The lack of a clear understanding of how glare induces discomfort (see Chapter 7) also makes the analysis and interpretation of problems attributed by VDT operators to glare difficult and uncertain. Nevertheless, several models and mathematical expressions for describing the effects of glare on visual comfort probability (VCP) have been formulated (see, e.g., Kaufman and Christensen, 1972). Extensive research dating from the 1920s (Holladay, 1926; Nowakowski, 1926) has provided the basis for such models. References to much of this research and other important issues related to discomfort glare are included in a report of the Commission Internationale de l'Eclairage (1980).

The report also includes a proposed CIE glare formula by H. D. Einhorn with a discussion of its rationale, quantitative aspects, and the significance and choice of scaling factors. The formula identifies the important variables and indicates how they are related:

$$CGI = 10 \log 0.1 \frac{(L^2 w)}{(p^2)} \times \frac{1 + E_d/500}{(E_e)}$$

where
CGI = CIE glare index (provisional name)
L   = Luminance of a glare source, in cd/m^2
w   = Solid angle of source, in steradian
P   = Guth position index
E_d = Direct vertical illuminance at eye due to all sources, in lux
E_e = Vertical illuminance at eye, in lux. E_e includes the indirect illuminance: $E_e = E_d + E_i$

The position index P is based on Luckiesh-Guth's research. For computer work it is best expressed as:

$$\frac{1}{P} = \frac{d^2 E}{d^2 + 1.5d + 4.6} + 0.12 (1-E)$$

with E = exp $(- 0.18 \, s^2/d + 0.011 \, s^3/d)$
where d = forward distance of source/height
      s = sideways distance of source-height (forward)
              means in the direction of the line of sight,
              sideways means perpendicular to it, height means
              height above eye level.)

In general, the higher the luminance of a glare source, the larger the source, the lower the background luminance, and the closer the source is to the line of sight, the greater is the capacity of the source to produce discomfort. The position index, P, is directional; a glare source located horizontally to the line of sight has greater potential for producing discomfort than an equivalent source located the same angular distance directly above the line of sight.

The use of comprehensive formulas of this type has not been reported in studies of VDTs. However, the potential for VDTs to induce discomfort glare can be estimated from reported luminance measurements and data from basic research on discomfort glare. Table 5.1 shows data (Guth, 1951) relating background luminance and glare-source size to glare-source luminance at the borderline between comfort and discomfort (BCD). Assuming that these data accurately represent discomfort glare thresholds for at least some VDT operators, it can be seen from Table 5.1 that some situations would induce discomfort. Fellmann and coworkers, using an illumination of 150 lux on eight different brands of VDTs, reported luminances ranging from 2-7 cd/m^2 for screen backgrounds, 8-110 cd/m^2 for consoles, and 8-45 cd/m^2 for keyboards (Fellmann et al., 1981). These values represent the background luminances (the approximate levels to which the operators would be adapted), that are best represented in the table by the 3.4 and 34 cd/m^2 values. Luminances in excess of 1,000 cd/m^2 from potential glare sources (e.g., windows and luminaires) have been measured in actual VDT workstations (Cakir et al., 1978; National Institute for Occupational Safety and Health, 1981). These values are glare source luminances. Values above the BCD values in the table would induce discomfort. (Note, however, that Guth used a flashing glare source. It is not clear how much the BCD values from steady sources in natural settings would differ. Eye movements and blinks would interrupt the retinal images of steady sources.) Several combinations of the measured or assumed conditions would produce discomfort glare.

A lighted environment that is properly designed and therefore comfortable for workers performing traditional desk-top tasks may not be comfortable for workers performing tasks involving VDTs for two reasons. First, the design of general office lighting assumes a depressed line of sight; however, when a VDT screen is viewed, the line of sight is at or near horizontal. The higher line of sight needed to view the screen brings ceiling luminaires closer to the line of sight, resulting in a higher glare index and a greater likelihood of discomfort glare. Second, the temporally and spatially averaged luminance is lower for positive-contrast VDTs, which results in a higher glare value.

TABLE 5.1 Borderline Between Comfort and Discomfort (BCD) Luminance for Intermittent Directly Viewed Glare Sources

	Diameter of Circular Glare Source (Degrees of Visual Angle)														
	0.66°			2.12°			5.72°			11.42°			22.62°		
	Background Luminance (cd/m²)														
	3.4	34	340	3.4	34	340	3.4	34	340	3.4	34	340	3.4	34	340
Glare source luminance at BCD (cd/m²)	2086	5740	15840	1072	2950	8144	548	1507	4156	291	805	2220	96	264	730
Luminance ratio	614	168	462	315	87	238	161	44	121	86	24	65	28.2	7.8	21

SOURCE: Guth (1951). Reprinted with permission from the Optical Society of America.

Glare problems have been reported in several studies involving VDTs. Although there are problems in the methods used and the interpretation of results in some of these studies (see Chapters 2 and 7 and Appendix A), there is little doubt that lighting and reflections were responsible for some of the reported operator complaints and problems.

A general analytic model for predicting task visibility under different lighting conditions may be useful in analyzing VDT task situations. This model is

$$VL = \tilde{C}_{ref} \times \frac{RCS}{0.0923} \times CRF \times DGF \times TAF$$

where (as defined in Commission Internationale de l'Eclairage, 1981):

VL =   Visibility level, a measure of the extent to which the equivalent contrast of a task visual display exceeds the visibility threshold of an observer for the same display at the same level of task background luminance, measured in units of the observer's threshold contrast.

$\tilde{C}_{ref}$ =   Reference equivalent contrast, the value of equivalent contrast of given task details under reference lighting.

RCS =   Relative contrast sensitivity, proportional values of contrast sensitivity expressed relative to the value obtained with a luminance of 100 cd/m^2.

CRF =   Contrast rendering factor, the measure of the visibility of a task in a real lighting installation in comparison with its visibility under reference lighting conditions, account being taken of lighting geometry and polarization of illuminance.

DGF =   Disability glare factor, a measure of a task in a given lighting installation in comparison with its visibility under reference lighting. The measure takes account of the two effects of the ocular stray light produced by the pattern of luminance in the surround of the task: (a) the reduction in image contrast, and (b) the increase in RCS due to visual adaptation to the sum of the focused light and stray light.

TAF =   Transient adaptation factor, a measure of task detail
         visibility in a given lighting installation in
         comparison with its visibility under reference
         lighting, account being taken of the transient
         adaptive effect that occurs when the eyes of the
         observer view luminances in the environment
         different from the task background luminance.

0.0923 = The value of the visibility threshold for the 4-minute
         disc task obtained by the reference observer at a
         level of task background luminance equal to 100
         cd/m^2.

This model is based on extensive laboratory data and has been used
in analyzing complex realistic visual performance, for example,
proofreading, visual search, and numerical verification. While it
has not yet been applied to VDT tasks, there is no obvious reason
why it should not be applied to such tasks. It incorporates several
factors, including transitional adaptation and disability glare
effects. Although this model has been criticized (see, e.g.,
Yonemura, 1977; Padmos and Vos, 1980) and may have important
limitations, it seems worthy of further validity tests, some of
which could include VDT applications.

Some aspects of an earlier version of the model incorporated a
visual discomfort formula (Commission Internationale de
l'Eclairage, 1975), and some recommended standards have been
used by Mayer and Barlier (1981) to evaluate 73 VDT workstations. Luminance measurements were made of screens,
keyboards, and documents. Contrasts of screen characters and
their backgrounds for 40 of the VDTs are plotted with CIE
visibility curves in Figure 5.3. Of the 40, 2 VDTs were above the
comfort limit; 3 were approximately at threshold (VL = 1), which
should make task performance very difficult or impossible; and 15
were in the range that would be expected to have a significant
effect on the performance of some tasks (VL < 8).

In summary, VDTs differ from objects and surfaces in non-VDT
workplaces because they usually have a highly specular, curved
glass surface in a more vertical plane. Consequently, workplaces
in which VDTs are used require lighting designs that differ from
those required in non-VDT workplaces. Lighting and equipment
arrangements that are appropriately designed for a particular task
and working situation should prevent glare and most other problems arising from lighting and reflections. Application of
established knowledge and principles of design in the field of
illuminating engineering can be expected to alleviate most of the
difficulties related to lighting and reflections in VDT-related work.

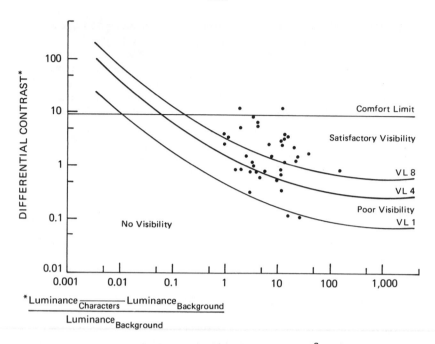

BACKGROUND LUMINANCE (cd/m^2)

FIGURE 5.3 Illuminating Engineering Society (IES) visual performance curve: visibility of screens. SOURCE: Mayer and Barlier (1981).

REVIEW OF VDT STUDIES

Field Surveys of VDT Workers

Several field surveys have attempted to determine the opinions of VDT operators regarding problems caused by lighting and reflections in the workplace. In some of these surveys, measurements of various aspects of the lighting conditions have also been made, and some investigators have attempted to relate those measurements to visual symptoms and complaints reported by VDT operators. Most of the surveys suffer from the kinds of limitations in method discussed in Chapter 2. Consequently, while the results of these surveys reveal that many VDT operators have complaints and symptoms related to workplace lighting conditions, they do not establish whether such complaints and symptoms are more frequent, more severe, or of a different nature than those that may be associated with non-VDT near-visual work. Our purpose in briefly reviewing several of these surveys is simply to provide an overview of the kinds of studies that have been conducted and the kinds of problems that have been reported.

There have been several published studies that used various types of questionnaires and interviews to determine the opinions of VDT operators about their work. In a study conducted by Ghiringelli (1980), 63 percent of operators reported that badly working equipment was a problem, 43 percent reported problems with reflections, and 43 percent also reported problems with "luminance." Using an unstructured interview technique, Grieco and coworkers (1980) interviewed an unspecified number of selected newspaper photocomposition VDT workers and reported that operators had problems with lighting, particularly with screen reflections. Dainoff (1980) and Dainoff and coworkers (1981) also used an unstructured interview technique in a study that covered 90 clerical workers, who reported that they worked with VTDs from 0-100 percent of the time (median 47 percent), and 31 data entry workers, who reported that they worked with VDTs 75 percent of the time. Complaints about lighting related specifically to the VDT were significantly higher in the data entry group; complaints about general workplace lighting, however, were made by the same percentage (37 percent) of workers in both groups. No attempt was made to relate complaints to specific aspects of the physical environment of the workplace. The designs of these studies do not permit an analysis of possible causal factors in reported complaints.

Several published studies present data on the types and frequency of complaints, accompanied by measurements of certain aspects of the lighting and reflection conditions. Hultgren and Knave (1974) studied an insurance office that had 17 VDTs at various locations in a room. A questionnaire was used to determine operator feelings about discomfort glare, eyestrain, and specific discomfort associated with reading the text on the screen. The luminance of the screen, illuminance of the work area, and angles of incident light and reflection were measured for 6 representative terminals. The operators reported problems with 13 of the 17 terminals in at least one of the three areas covered by the questionnaire. The luminance ratio of the screen to the brightest region in the immediate vicinity of the screen was a maximum of 1:500. In the worst case, reflected images had double or triple the luminance of an area of the screen containing a character. The character luminance was not measured directly. This study involved such a small sample that firm conclusions about the relationship between complaints and the VDT environment cannot be drawn. It did indicate, however, that operators in this one location had problems with glare.

Cakir and coworkers (1978) conducted a field study of 30 companies in which more than 1,000 VDT operators participated. Statements from operators about lighting problems were obtained by means of a questionnaire, and various aspects of the lighted environment were measured. The authors reported that the luminaires providing the general room lighting were a source of operator complaints. Luminaires of different construction elicited significant response differences to a question concerning direct glare. Bare fluorescent lamps were complained about more frequently as a source of direct glare than were luminaires constructed with some type of diffusing cover. Operators also rated bare fluorescent lamps as poorest with regard to the visibility of screen characters. More than 50 percent of the workers reported seeing reflections in their screens and, again, bare fluorescent lamps were singled out by the operators as producing more problems with screen reflections than luminaires with diffusing covers.

At selected sites and on selected VDTs, Cakir and coworkers measured the luminances of ceilings, luminaires, display documents, keyboards, and screen backgrounds. Ceiling luminances ranged between 15 and 35 cd/m^2, while luminaires in the ceilings had luminances over 1,000 cd/m^2. Luminance ratios between screen background and display documents were found to be 1:6 if no antireflection filter was used over the VDT screen and 1:100 if a filter was used. The luminance ratio between the screen and the keyboard ranged from 2:1 to 1:70. Problems with beat frequencies, which might arise from the flicker of fluorescent lights and the refresh rate of the VDT screen, were not found.

On the basis of the responses to a questionnaire, Elias and coworkers (1979, 1980) determined that 70 percent of operators who worked in an office that had windows almost all the way around had complaints about general lighting, while 45 percent of those who worked in an office with fewer windows had such complaints. The tasks differed in the two offices--in the windowed office the task was predominantly data entry;[1] in the other office the task was interactive—and so did complaints about reflections on the screens: 45 percent of the data entry group and 65 percent of the interactive group had such complaints. The authors ascribe the higher frequency of complaints about screen reflections in the interactive group to the greater period of time these operators viewed the screen. The two groups also differed in complaints

[1]Elias and coworkers (1980) define the task as "data acquisition"; however, the description of the task (Elias et al., 1979) corresponds more closely to what is referred to in this report as data entry (see Chapter 1).

about glare: 80 percent of the data entry operators and 52 percent of the interactive operators reported complaints related to glare that occurred, "sometimes" or "often" (four responses were available: "often," "sometimes," "rarely," "never"). The authors ascribe the greater number of glare complaints in the data entry group to various factors, including range of contrast.

Luminance levels were measured at a typical worksite in the data entry (windowed) office. The luminance ratio between the screen and the document was 1:8.5; between the screen and its periphery, the maximum ratio was 1:500, with daylight from a window providing general illumination on a sunny day; when illumination was provided only by a luminaire, the luminance ratio was 1:108. A higher percentage of data entry than of interactive operators reported discomfort glare. The authors ascribed this finding to the higher frequency of measured saccadic eye movements between objects of disparate luminances made by the data entry operators.

Stewart (1980a) assessed environmental problems at 80 VDT workplaces. The most frequently occuring environmental problem was thermal (100 percent of the workplaces), but the next most frequently occurring problems were glare (71 percent of the workplaces) and reflections from windows and luminaires (83 percent of the workplaces). Measured illumination levels at the workplaces ranged from 100 to 2,500 lux.

A study conducted under the auspices of the New Zealand Department of Health at selected VDT workplaces showed that screen reflections occurred on 42 percent of the VDTs surveyed (Coe et al., 1980). No statistical relationship between room lighting intensity and presence of screen reflections was found. Of the workplaces sampled, approximately one-third exceeded a 3:1 ratio of luminances between hard copy and screen, and more than half exceeded that ratio between the immediate background of the screen and the screen itself. For those VDT tasks requiring hard copy, 54 percent of the operators viewing hard copy illumi-nated with less than 250 lux reported asthenopia (sore eyes and visual discomfort), 55 percent of the operators viewing hard copy illuminated between 250 and 500 lux reported asthenopia, and 34 percent of the operators whose hard copy was illuminated with more than 500 lux reported asthenopia. A comparison group was used in this study, but no data are reported on lighting complaints of the non-VDT comparison group.

Field Surveys Comparing VDT and Non-VDT Work

The studies reviewed above indicate that lighting and reflections do cause problems for VDT workers; however, these problems may not be unique to VDT use, but may be present in general office work. Without evaluating non-VDT work, no comparisons can be made regarding such complaints in VDT and non-VDT tasks. Two studies have attempted such comparisons.

Laubli and coworkers (1980) conducted a field study in which illumination and luminance levels were measured at workstations used in four different types of office tasks: (1) data entry VDT work; (2) interactive VDT work; (3) traditional clerical work; and (4) typing. At 90 percent of the VDT workstations, the illumination levels of source documents were between 100 and 1,900 lux; at workstations used for traditional clerical work or typing, the levels were between 100 and 3,200 lux. The luminance ratios between source document and screen background ranged from 7:1 to 87:1 at VDT workstations. The frequency of ocular and visual symptoms--pains, burning, fatigue, shooting pain, red eyes, headaches, blurring of near and far vision, flicker vision, and double images (all referred to as eye impairments in the study)-- increased as luminance ratios increased. The incidence of symptoms was highest in the interactive VDT operators; it was lower in data entry VDT operators and in typists (and approximately the same for these two groups), and considerably lower for workers performing traditional clerical work. Although images reflected by the VDT screen had lower luminances than screen characters, the measured intensity of the reflections was correlated with reported annoyance; it was not, however, correlated with frequency of ocular or visual symptoms.

Stammerjohn and coworkers (1981) conducted a study at four newspapers and one insurance company. At selected workstations, they measured illuminances and luminances in operators' general visual field, including the luminance of the screen background, but not that of the display characters. Subjective operator ratings on a five-point scale from "no bother or problem" to "constantly bothersome" were obtained on screen brightness, character brightness, readability, screen angle, keyboard angle, screen height, keyboard height, distance to the screen, distance to the keyboard, screen glare, keyboard glare, noise from the VDT, and screen flicker.

The majority of workstations had illuminances between 500 and 700 lux, with a low of 300 and a high of 1,200 lux. The range of luminance ratios in the immediate visual field of the operators was from 1:2 to 1:60. Potential glare sources (windows, luminaires) were reported at 46 of the 53 workstations. Luminances of these sources were near 2,100 cd/m^2. Reflected glare from windows or overhead lights was present on most of the screens surveyed at one site. Luminances of the reflected images had maxima of 3-60 cd/m^2. Although character luminance was not measured, the investigators had difficulty in reading the screen text from VDTs that had particularly high reflected glare levels (17 percent of those examined).

Several aspects of the VDTs were reported as bothersome by operators: screen glare (85 percent), character brightness (70 percent), readability (69 percent), flicker (68 percent), and screen brightness (62 percent). A slight majority were satisfied with workstation and background illumination. However, 80 percent of the VDT operators reported trouble with glare from the workstation lighting. More than 60 percent of the non-VDT operators also reported problems with glare from workstation lighting.

Because of employee anonymity involving the use of the questionnaires, specific complaints cannot be related to specific VDTs and therefore to specific design features. This study did, however, determine that a significant relationship exists between complaints regarding visual function and employee rating of workplace design parameters, including glare, screen angle, noise from the VDT, and screen flicker.

Laboratory Studies

In a laboratory investigation, Radl (1980) demonstrated the importance to operator comfort and to one measure of performance of graded luminance from the screen to its surround. The subjects had to transcribe letters from the screen to a paper sheet. They viewed a VDT screen with a background luminance of 18 cd/m^2 and symbol luminance of 120 cd/m^2 with a surround of 4,200 cd/m^2 (i.e., a glare source) encompassing about 75 degrees of the subjects' visual field. The initial experiments used a black frame of varying dimensions around the VDT screen. The results are summarized in Table 5.2. Radl also compared the effects of positive and negative contrast on performance of the same task and on rating of visual comfort, using 24 subjects. The subjects rated negative contrast (dark characters on a light background) as more comfortable (general illumination of 500 lux; screen surround not described), and performance was also greater with this presentation. Both findings were reported as statistically significant.

Bauer and Cavonius (1980) examined the differential effects of positive and negative contrast on performance of a letter identification task. The display presentations were (1) low-luminance, positive contrast (10 cd/m^2 background), (2) high-luminance positive contrast (80 cd/m^2 background), and (3) negative contrast (80 cd/m^2 background). The error rate was lowest for the negative-contrast display and highest for the high-luminance positive-contrast display.

TABLE 5.2   Graded Luminance and Operator Performance and Comfort

Width of Frame	Performance(%)[a]	Rated Visual Comfort (Worst, 0; Best, 7)
No frame	42	0.32
7°	67	1.45
11°	69	1.80
16°	84	2.05
21°	63	3.07
11°[b]	85	3.15

[a] Relative to performance tested in the absence of glare.
[b] Frame continuously shaded from black at the screen to white at the outer edge.

In a second experiment, Bauer and Cavonius (1980) compared the speed and accuracy of subjects using positive- or negative-contrast displays in detecting discrepancies between a VDT presentation and a typewritten presentation. The two conditions compared were positive-contrast display (symbol luminance 40–65 cd/m^2, screen background luminance < 10 cd/m^2, ambient illumination 270 lux) and negative-contrast display (symbol luminance set as low as possible, screen background luminance 50–70 cd/m^2, ambient illumination 550 lux). The negative-contrast display produced the fewest errors and fastest performance time, and 18 of the 19 subjects preferred the negative contrast; the one subject who preferred positive contrast actually performed better on the negative-contrast display. As noted in Chapter 4, both the Bauer and Cavonius (1980) study and the Radl (1980) study should be interpreted cautiously because changes in contrast polarity were combined with changes in ambient illumination and absolute contrast magnitude.

In summary, the field surveys and a few limited laboratory studies of VDT-related work indicate that workers who use VDTs have problems caused by lighting and reflections. However, we found no studies that compared equivalent, appropriately illuminated and arranged VDT- and non-VDT tasks and working situations, and so we cannot draw conclusions about the relative number, types, and severity of complaints and problems related to lighting and reflections in VDT and non-VDT work.

6
Anthropometry and Biomechanics in VDT Applications

Biomechanics and anthropometry play important roles in the design of VDT workstations. They are intertwined with other ergonomic aspects of the workplace and have implications for both postural and visual task requirements. A classic example of the way in which visual and postural aspects are interlinked is that of an operator who has to bend his or her head back in order to read the screen through the lower part of bifocals. Adapting this posture can cause neck and back pain and possibly visual discomfort and reduction in performance. Similarly, the positions of the keyboard, source document, and screen all have implications for visual accommodation. If the ambient illumination level is raised to enhance the legibility of a source document, the legibility of the characters on the screen may decrease.

Since only relatively little adaptation can be expected from human operators, the technical elements of a VDT system must be selected to fit the operator. In fact, all system components, that is, the display, the workplace furniture, the environment, and the work tasks and schedules must be fitted to each other, and all of them to the operator: none of these components can be considered independently.

Human factors problems can be analyzed in a systems context. Two major systems are involved in VDT applications: the job and the operator. The job may be divided into two subsystems, workstation design and task characteristics, both of which impose certain demands on the operator. The other major system, the operator, may also be thought of in terms of two subsystems: biomechanical/anthropometric factors and personal factors. Unless the proper balance between job demands and operator capabilities is established, there may be adverse health consequences, as indicated by physical complaints and symptoms, absenteeism, and so forth. Problems must be studied at the level of subsystems (e.g, investigating biomechanical and anthropometric factors) to obtain information sufficiently detailed to propose practical solutions.

This chapter addresses anthropometry and biomechanics in VDT applications and the ways in which they influence appropriate design of workstations, particularly the choice of chairs, support stands for keyboard and display tables, footrests, wristrests, armrests, and document holders. The first part of this chapter reviews several field surveys of postural strain in VDT work. The second part reviews and analyzes the anthropometric, biomechanical, and physiological factors that influence the appropriate design of VDT workstations. The implications of this analysis for the design of VDT tasks and workstations are discussed in Chapter 9.

POSTURAL STRAIN

Of the substantial body of literature on the postural strain associated with VDT work, nearly all is based on subjective reports of muscular discomfort. Some researchers support this data with medical observations or measurements of body angles, chair and table heights, and viewing distances. Overall, the research represents an attempt to isolate VDT design problems, but because of problems in the methodologies of many studies, the results are difficult to interpret.

Practically all of the research has been performed in the field, using existing groups of subjects. The main sample has always consisted of VDT operators; in some cases investigators classified the operators by their tasks, such as data entry, data acquisition, or interactive work. Approximately one-half of the studies have used a non-VDT comparison group.

Several problems are inherent in survey research using static group comparisons (see Chapter 2). For example, by sensitizing subjects to the issues under investigation, surveys tend to be reactive. Surveys may also be influenced by uncontrolled psychosocial factors. For example, one study (Smith et al., 1980; National Institute for Occupational Safety and Health, 1981) found that, depending on job demands and task requirements, different types of health problems were reported. Workers who were allowed more flexibility and autonomy generally voiced complaints of a psychological nature, such as anxiety and irritability, while workers whose jobs were rigid and offered little control reported more visual and musculoskeletal problems. The authors mentioned that union negotiations at the time of the survey may have influenced the results. Task characteristics, psychosocial factors, and personal characteristics influence the reporting of symptoms; the results of survey research studies must, therefore, be interpreted very carefully.

Table 6.1 summarizes six studies that reported subjective data on pains in various parts of the body and in which the VDT group was compared with a non-VDT group (but see the discussion in Chapter 2 regarding comparisons between VDT and non-VDT groups). Since the studies used different methods or questions, or both, the percentages in the table can be compared only within each study. As shown in the table, two studies indicate that VDT operators reported more symptoms than non-VDT operators (Arndt, 1981; and Smith et al., 1981). The study by Eisen (1981) showed mixed results. In the study by Hunting and coworkers (1981), traditional office workers had fewer complaints than data entry and interactive VDT users and typists (except for leg pains, for which data entry workers had many more reports than the other three groups). Finally, Coe and coworkers (1980) found only differences by sex: females reported more problems than males, which was also found by Onishi and coworkers (1973).

OVERVIEW OF BIOMECHANICAL FACTORS

Work Posture

When a person stands upright, the body's center of gravity is located in the upper part of the pelvis, vertically above the arch of the foot. Any movement of the trunk, head, or arms requires a compensating countermove by the pelvis. For example, if the arms are extended forward, the hips will move backward. In this way the body redistributes its weight and achieves balance. In some postures, such as sitting and lying down, balance is maintained with only modest contributions of certain groups of muscles. In others, there may be a great deal of effort, with static muscle contractions required. Most of the physiological changes associated with postural stress are caused by static muscle contractions (Troup, 1978).

Posture, implying a more or less static condition, is found in few natural biological systems. Most systems in the body are in a dynamic equilibrium, with continuous changes around an average value. Troup (1978) emphasized that it is generally easy to relieve symptoms of postural stress simply by moving around. Kramer (1973) observed that such postural changes result in a massaging action of the discs in the spine. Branton and Grayson (1967) studied train passengers and found that there were cyclic postural changes, which they interpreted as necessary to prevent postural strain. Ostrom (1981) pointed out that "dynamic sitting," implying a change in posture about every five minutes, is important for comfort and promotes good circulation.

The design of a VDT workstation should make it easy to change work postures. For example, a flat seat pan is better than an

TABLE 6.1   Percentage of Various Populations Reporting Body Pains

Author and Groups Investigated	Pain Location						
	Head	Neck	Arms	Wrists	Back (General)	Lumbar	Legs
Coe et al. (1980)							
VDT users	32						
Input	45						
Creative	20						
Editing	41						
Dialogue	18						
Non-VDT	41						
VDT users							
Male	19						
Female	40						
Non-VDT							
Male	22						
Female	49						
Arndt (1981)							
VDT users	65[a]						
Non-VDT	39[a]						
Eisen (1981)							
VDT users							
Mainly editing		75[b]	27	7	76		24
Non-VDT		75[b]	38	19	66		34
Hunting et al. (1981)							
VDT users							
Data entry		11			9	9	13
Dialogue		5			6	11	6
Non-VDT							
Typists		6			9	10	5
Traditional office work		1			2	2	6
Smith et al. (1981)							
VDT users							
Clerical		56[b]	37		78		
Non-VDT		19[b]	20		56		

[a] Head and neck pain.
[b] Neck and shoulder pain.

"anatomical seat pan," molded after the contours of the posterior, because the latter inhibits movements (Vernon, 1924). Adjustable or flexible provisions at the VDT workstation, such as a detachable keyboard, a movable document holder, and an adjustable chair allow movements and are therefore important in preventing postural stress.

Muscular Load

There is an important distinction between dynamic work and static contraction of muscles. Dynamic work is characterized by a rhythmic change of contraction and relaxation of the muscles, which is favorable for blood circulation. Static effort, on the other hand, is characterized by sustained contraction, such as brought about by static postures. During static efforts, blood flow through the involved muscles is impaired (due to contracted muscles and blocked blood vessels) and waste products (e.g., lactic acid) accumulate (Astrand and Rodahl, 1977). This condition may cause acute pain in the statically loaded muscle. Excessive static loads may also lead to rheumatic diseases that affect the joints, ligaments, and tendons and to the development of arthrosis of an inflammatory and degenerative nature (van Wely, 1970). The peritendinitus that frequently occurs in the lower arm of typists is caused by excessive static load (Tichauer, 1976).

Static workloads can often be alleviated by providing suitable body supports, such as armrests on chairs and wristrests in front of keyboards. A recent innovation is the split keyboard, the halves of which are located on inclined surfaces that provide forearm support.

Joint Angles

Every joint has a limited range of movement (Grieco et al., 1978). The closer the joint's position approaches either of its extremes, the more uncomfortable the position becomes. Therefore, work activities should be performed with the joints in about the middle of their range of movement. This is particularly important for the joints of the neck, trunk, and upper limbs (van Wely, 1970).

Two common examples of poor posture caused by working near the limits of joint ranges of movement are the VDT operator with presbyopia who bends his or her head back in order to observe the screen through the lower part of bifocals and the outward angling of the hands (ulnar deviation) in VDT operators and typists. The standard keyboard with horizontal rows of keys requires an extreme inward rotation of the hands (pronation). Lateral down-tilt of each half of a split keyboard may alleviate the static muscle tension required to maintain this position (Kroemer, 1972; Grandjean et al., 1981).

When a person moves from a standing to a sitting position, the hip angle decreases from 180° to 90°. Anatomically, this movement is fairly complicated; about 60° of the bending takes place in the hip joint, and the remaining 30° is due to the flattening of the lumbar curve. Thus, while sitting, the lordosis (forward bend) of the lumbar spine is flattened out. Most of the angular change takes place in the fourth and fifth lumbar discs (Schobert, 1962). Since these discs are involved in many lower back problems, it is important to supply chairs with lumbar supports. Keegan (1953) pointed out that the angular change in the lumbar region when repositioning from a standing to a sitting posture starts when the hip angle reaches about 135°. This angle corresponds to a resting position (commonly assumed while sleeping) for which the muscles of the front of the thighs (quadriceps and iliacus) and the muscles underneath the leg (hamstring) are in relaxed balance.

It is also important to provide seats that allow operators to bend their knees since the decrease in lumbar lordosis while sitting is further emphasized if a seated person stretches his or her leg. Stretched legs cause a rotation of the pelvis due to the pull action of the hamstring muscle.

Sitting brings the ischial tuberosities (the rounded arches of bone at the base of the pelvis) close to the skin. This can be felt by placing a hand between the body and the seat. The bony protrusions absorb most of the sitting pressure (Applied Ergonomics, 1970). Pressure between the body and the seat can be changed by assuming various postures, such as crossing one's legs, propping an arm on a table or armrest, or leaning forward or back in the chair. For distribution of pressure, the seat should be firmly upholstered, neither too soft nor too hard. Nerves can be stimulated and blood flow restricted if there is pressure on body tissue, which may happen if there is not enough space for the leg between the seat and the table. It can also occur if the edge of the seat cuts into the underpart of the knee. The seat edge must, therefore, be well rounded, and there must be clearance for an operator's legs. The more often major or minor adjustments of posture are made, the less likely is discomfort.

Many of the complaints of VDT operators refer to sustained postures of the neck, shoulders, upper and lower extremities, and trunk. If operators had free choices they would probably move around, stand in different locations, and sit in various relaxed or upright positions. Choice of different postures, static and dynamic, would certainly alleviate many of the physical and psychological problems found with the confined seated position required at many VDT workstations.

With current VDT technology, the eyes must remain in a rather fixed location relative to the display, the hands must be kept over the keyboard, and the feet are confined to the open space under the table or support. Hence, only a limited choice of postures is available to an operator, and the chair should therefore allow various and easy adjustments in its dimensions and angulations. In some instances it might be feasible and desirable for an operator to change between seated and standing positions. To accommodate a person either sitting or standing at the same workstation would obviously require a rather elaborate workplace design. One can, however, often provide an extra workstation designed for standing operation, which may be used occasionally for a change of posture. Ergonomic data for sit/stand workstations are available (see U.S. Department of Defense, 1971, 1974, 1981; Ayoub and Halcomb, 1976; Woodson, 1981).

Anthropometry

Body dimensions of the user population are of primary importance for the design of the VDT workstation. The composition of the working population of the United States is changing dramatically. More women are entering occupations traditionally dominated by males and vice versa. These changes must be considered when designing furniture and other equipment for VDT workstations.

Most existing anthropometric data for the U.S. population apply to various military populations and cannot be readily used for estimating body dimensions of the working population. Since the military population is a subsample of the entire population, civilian body dimensions have recently been extrapolated from data on military populations. McConville and coworkers (1981) matched individuals from civilian and military samples in stature and weight creating a subsample of the military population that represents civilians on these two dimensions. From this subsample, dimensions other than height and weight were selected and compared to civilian data. For males, there was excellent fit: 99 percent of all civilians could be matched with a member of the military. For females the attempt was less successful, but 94 percent of the civilians could be matched. Though not complete, the data represent the most current compilation of body dimensions for the U.S civilian population (see Table 6.2).

In anthropometric investigations a person is measured in a standardized erect/sitting position with joint angles at 0°, 90°, or 180°. Each of these is referred to as an "anatomical position." Unfortunately, this method does not provide functional dimensions that describe the continuously changing positions of a human body. Until better translation techniques are developed to

TABLE 6.2 U.S. Civilian Body Dimensions, Female/Male, for Ages 20 to 60 Years

Body Dimension (cm)	Percentiles			Standard Deviation
	5th	50th	95th	
Stature (height)	149.5/161.8	160.5 /173.6	171.3/184.4	6.6 /6.9
Eye height	138.3/151.1	148.9 /162.4	159.3/172.7	6.4 /6.6[a]
Shoulder (acromion) height	121.1/132.3	131.1 /142.8	141.9/152.4	6.3 /6.1[a]
Elbow height	93.6/100.0	101.2 /109.9	108.8/119.0	4.6 /5.8[a]
Knuckle height	64.3/ 69.8	70.2 / 75.4	75.9/ 80.4	3.5 /3.2[a]
Height, sitting	78.6/ 84.2	85.0 / 90.6	90.7/ 96.7	3.5 /3.7
Eye height, sitting	67.5/ 72.6	73.3 / 78.6	78.5/ 84.4	3.3 /3.6[a]
Shoulder height, sitting	49.2/ 52.7	55.7 / 59.4	61.7/ 65.8	3.8 /4.0[a]
Elbow rest height, sitting	18.1/ 19.0	23.3 / 24.3	28.1/ 29.4	2.9 /3.0
Knee height, sitting	45.2/ 49.3	49.8 / 54.3	54.4/ 59.3	2.7 /2.9
Popliteal height, sitting	35.5/ 39.2	39.8 / 44.2	44.3/ 48.8	2.6 /2.8
Thigh clearance height, sitting	10.6/ 11.4	13.7 / 14.4	17.5/ 17.7	1.8 /1.7
Head breadth	13.6/ 14.4	14.5 / 15.4	15.5/ 16.4	0.57/0.59

Head circumference	52.2/ 53.8	54.9 / 56.8	57.7/ 59.3	1.63/1.68
Interpupillary distance	5.1/ 5.5	5.83/ 6.20	6.5/ 6.8	0.44/0.39
Forward reach, functional	64.0/ 76.3	71.0 / 82.5	79.0/ 88.3	4.5 /3.6[a]
Elbow-fingertip length	38.5/ 44.1	42.1 / 47.9	46.0/ 51.4	2.2 /2.2[a]
Hand length	16.4/ 17.6	17.95/ 19.05	19.8/ 20.6	1.04/0.93
Hand breadth, metacarpal	7.0/ 8.2	7.66/ 8.88	8.4/ 9.8	0.41/0.47
Hand circumference, metacarpal	16.9/ 19.9	18.36/ 21.55	19.9/ 23.5	0.80/1.09
Chest depth	21.4/ 21.4	24.2 / 24.2	29.7/ 27.6	2.5 /1.9[a]
Elbow-to-elbow breadth	31.5/ 35.0	38.4 / 41.7	49.1/ 50.6	5.4 /4.6
Hip breadth, sitting	31.2/ 30.8	36.4 / 35.4	43.7/ 40.6	3.7 /2.8
Buttock-knee length, sitting	51.8/ 54.0	56.9 / 59.4	62.5/ 64.2	3.1 /3.0
Foot length	22.3/ 24.8	24.1 / 26.9	26.2/ 29.0	1.19/1.28
Foot breadth	8.1/ 9.0	8.84/ 9.79	9.7/ 10.7	0.50/0.53
Weight (kg)	46.2/ 56.2	61.1 / 74.0	89.9/ 97.1	13.8 /12.6

[a] Estimate.

SOURCE: Kroemer (1981). Reprinted with permission from the American Institute of Industrial Engineers, Inc., 25 Technology Park/Atlanta, Norcross, GA 30092.

convert static anthropometric measures to functional dimensions, the following guidelines might be used to design a VDT workstation:

1. Stature, sitting height, eye height, and shoulder height should be reduced by 3 to 5 percent from the erect sitting measures (Brown and Schaum, 1980; Kroemer and Price, 1982).

2. For comfortable reach, forward and lateral reach should be decreased by 30 percent from the erect sitting measures.

3. Popliteal height, knee height, and elbow height should not be changed from the standard positions.

The simplest design model is the "average person" (50th percentile). Unfortunately, even one person who is average in many or all body measures is extremely hard to find. It was shown three decades ago by Daniels (1952) that simultaneous use of several average measures is false and results in a design that fits nobody well. Other misleading assumptions are that a large female can be represented by the body dimensions of an average male and that the dimensions of a small male are similar to those of an average female.

It is becoming standard practice to design to accommodate 90 percent of the population, disregarding the upper and lower 5 percent. For this reason, anthropometric data are often expressed in terms of 5th, 50th, and 95th percentile measures. These concepts are described in Table 6.3. Since body measurements usually have a normal distribution, any percentile measure can be derived from the values of the mean ($\bar{x}$) and the standard deviation (S.D.). Anthropometric tables are available for males and females. For mixed civilian populations (e.g., 20 percent male and 80 percent female), there are special formulas for the calculation of percentiles (see Roebuck et al., 1975 and Kroemer, 1982).

WORKSTATION DESIGN

Effects of Chair Design Features on the Spine

Several studies have analyzed how pressure in lumbar discs and electromyographic (EMG) potentials from the muscles in the lower back are affected by various sitting postures (Nachemson and Elfstron, 1970; Andersson and Ortengren, 1974, 1979). Disc pressure was measured by inserting a needle with a strain-gauge measuring device into the third lumbar disc, and the EMG was recorded using skin electrodes. The investigations showed that disc pressure and EMG potentials were considerably less for standing than for sitting, with or without support. Simultaneous

TABLE 6.3　50th, 95th, and 5th Percentile Anthropometric
Measures

Percentile	Description
50th	Average value of body dimension ($\bar{x}$); 50% of the population is smaller
95th	95% of the population is smaller; can be calculated from the formula $\bar{x} + 1.65$ S.D.[a]
5th	5% of the population is smaller; can be calculated from the formula $\bar{x} - 1.65$ S.D.

[a] S.D. is standard deviation.

X-ray investigations showed that the lordosis of the lumbar region decreased by an average of 38° when subjects sat down. The highest pressure was obtained for a person lifting a weight, and the lowest pressure was obtained during a relaxed, reclining position. It should be noted that typing (without wrist support) induced disc pressures far higher than ordinary handwriting activities in which forearms were supported. Disc pressures decreased monotonically with backrest inclination and the size of the lumbar support. Complementary investigations showed that a seat inclination of 6° towards the back decreased disc pressure in comparison with a horizontal seat.

Summarizing these investigations, Andersson and Ortengren (1979) pointed out that there was 35 percent more disc pressure while sitting than while standing. When the backrest inclination increased from 80° to 130°, the pressure decreased by about 50 percent. An increase in lumbar support to +4 cm decreased pressure by 30 percent. The maximum combined decrease due to simultaneous change in backrest angle and lumbar support was 65 percent.

These findings support the notions that the optimum seat back angle is about 110°-120°, that a suitable backward inclination of the seat pan is about 15°, and that there should be a pronounced lumbar support from the seat back (Kroemer, 1971; Yamaguchi et al., 1972; Andersson and Ortengren, 1974; Grandjean, 1980). However, different design solutions have also been proposed. Staffel (1889), for example, maintained that the seat should have a forward slope. This opinion was recently supported by Mandal (1981), who reported that lordosis of the lumbar spine is maintained if the seat surface is tilted 20° forward, which increases the hip angle to about 120°. The resulting seating postures are quite unusual.

Adjustability of the seat height is considered mandatory in most VDT design guidelines (Helander, 1981). Since people differ in size and postural preferences, adjustability of the equipment appears necessary despite the fact that few experiments have been done to quantify how desirable and how necessary it is. McLeod and coworkers (1980) performed an experiment with chair height and backrest height adjusted in three different combinations, all used with the same desks. Overall, a medium setting was perceived as most comfortable. (Interestingly, the subjects thought the desk heights were manipulated and not the chair adjustments; this also supports the notion that system components interact with each other.) Another study observed the adjustments in seat and backrest height actually made by VDT users in a new library. Of those responding to a questionnaire, 30 percent adjusted their seat height and 35 percent the back support. Both studies concluded that maladjusted seating produces negative effects. There are obviously trade-offs among the benefits of adjustability and its cost. The actual use of adjustable features depends on the user population, the task, and on the ease of adjustment.

Effects of Working Height on Postural Strain

Choice of the working height of the hands, and associated arm and trunk postures, is among the most controversial design aspects for keyboard work. Lundervold (1951) quoted three contradictory schools of thought indicating that the working height should be such that a keyboard operator (typist) can work with the elbows at about 90°, with the forearms sloping downward, or with the forearms sloping upward. These recommendations have obvious effects on the height of the keyboard and its support stand and also on the seat height to be selected.

The first recommendation, having the elbows at right angles and the upper arms hanging vertically, is reflected in the proposed German regulation for VDT operators (Helander, 1981). Assuming a knee angle of 90° and the thighs about horizontal (as is the usual recommendation found in the literature in order to achieve a "correct" sitting height), an extremely thin table top and a very thin keyboard must be used to allow the right angle at the elbow, with the upper arm hanging vertically. As Table 6.2 indicates, the average differences between elbow rest height and the upper side of the thigh are between 10 cm and 13 cm. In order to allow sufficient height of the open leg room, the table top and keyboard combined cannot be thicker than about 10 cm. With such a small margin, the relative height adjustments of chair and keyboard support must be very fine.

Recent studies raise questions about the appropriateness of the 90° elbow recommendations. Zipp and coworkers (1980) measured

EMG in several muscles during a typing task. They concluded that EMG increases with increasing elbow angle, and they found a flat minimum in EMG activities for angles between 90° and 75°. These measurements do not support the idea that the forearms should slope downwards (i.e., that the elbow angle should be larger than 90°); furthermore, such a posture would leave almost no room between thighs and hand position, which would make it difficult to accommodate a suitable keyboard without infringing on needed leg space.

The findings of Zipp and coworkers are supported by those of Grandjean and coworkers,[1] who found that typists generally preferred to elevate the forearms, that is, to decrease the elbow angle, when they were provided with divided keyboards and wrist supports. Furthermore, various studies show that the upper arms are not usually hanging down vertically, but are slightly elevated both sagitally and frontally. In the Grandjean and coworkers study, subjects used a chair with a high backrest that allowed them to lean back fully and comfortably. This is indicative, again, of the various interactions between components of workstation and work habits.

Effects of Display Position on Postural Strain

Human engineering guidelines agree on a preferred downward slope of the line of sight of from 15° to 30° (Cakir et al., 1980; Rupp, 1981; U.S. Department of Defense, 1981). Consequently, the center of the display should be distinctly lower than a VDT operator's eyes. The height difference depends on the declination of the line of sight, α, against the horizontal, and on the preferred viewing distance, D:

$$\Delta H = D \sin \alpha$$

Both the preferred viewing distance and the preferred declination are highly subjective. For example, Grandjean and coworkers[2] reported (for their special experimental conditions) that their subjects preferred angles of between 4° and 14°. This finding indicates a need for further research.

It should be noted in this context that the optical correction for near-work routinely provided presbyopic individuals is likely to be at an inappropriate distance for reading a VDT screen. Multi-

---

[1] Etienne Grandjean, Swiss Federal Institute of Technology, Zurich, personal communicaton, January 1982.
[2] See footnote 1.

focal lenses may not be designed to allow a person to view a VDT screen through the segment for near work without tilting his or her head to an uncomfortable level.

It is obvious that many traditional exhortations and recommendations are somewhat questionable in the light of current knowledge. For example, people should not and will not "sit straight and upright"--if the location of the hands and the screen, the use of glasses (even with inappropriate lenses), and the availability of a good back support prompt or allow other postures. A modern workseat allows good support and a relaxed seating posture that uses a full backrest and permits an operator to lean back. This is likely to bring about a working height slightly above elbow rest height (measured while sitting). This in turn allows a relatively high open leg room when thin support stand surfaces and keyboards are used.

Different operators will select different postures and adjustments of workstation components, and the latter are dependent on each other. Furthermore, experience has shown that the ease of adjustment will determine whether the workplace components will be adapted to each other and whether individual comfort and postural satisfaction can be achieved. It is apparent that much adjustability in all major workstation components is necessary to allow individual accommodation according to body size, postural preferences, and work habits.

7
Visual Tasks, Functions, and Symptoms

This chapter addresses several interrelated questions: Are the visual complaints of VDT workers qualitatively or quantitatively different from those of non-VDT workers performing comparable near-visual tasks? What aspects of VDT work and non-VDT work might influence visual symptoms? Are there unique features of VDT equipment or job tasks that affect the comfort and visual performance of workers? What does the often-used term "visual fatigue" mean, and does it represent a useful concept?

VISUAL ISSUES IN VDT STUDIES

Field Surveys

Visual Complaints

Field surveys of the vision of VDT workers have received widespread attention in both popular literature (e.g., New York Committee for Occupational Safety and Health, 1980; Working Women, National Association of Office Workers, 1980; DeMatteo et al., 1981; Working Women Education Fund, 1981) and technical literature (e.g., Grandjean and Vigliani, 1980) and have been the basis for concern about the well-being of VDT workers. A majority of surveys have reported that more than 50 percent of VDT workers indicated that they at least occasionally experienced some type of ocular discomfort (irritation, pain, or fatigue involving the eyes) or blurring or flickering of vision (Cakir et al., 1978; Gunnarsson and Soderberg, 1979; Coe et al., 1980; Elias et al., 1980; Gunnarsson and Soderberg, 1980; Rey and Meyer, 1980; Smith et al., 1980; Arndt et al., 1981; National Institute for Occupational Safety and Health, 1981; Sauter et al., 1981; Smith et al., 1981). In studies that included comparison groups of non-VDT workers, a majority have reported that complaints related to vision were more prevalent in the VDT subjects (Laubli et al., 1980; Rey and Meyer, 1980; Smith et al., 1980, 1981; Arndt et al., 1981; National Institute for Occupational Safety and Health, 1981; Sauter et al., 1981). Coe and coworkers (1980) reported that while the prevalence of fatiguelike effects of visual discomfort was higher in VDT workers than in comparison groups, the prevalence of irritantlike effects and other subjective eye complaints was similar in the two groups.

Some surveys have reported that the prevalence of complaints of ocular discomfort increased with increasing percentage of work time spent working with VDTs (Rey and Meyer, 1980; Dainoff et al., 1981) and was higher in full-time than in part-time workers (Coe et al., 1980). Some studies have reported that the prevalence of complaints varied with the type of VDT work performed (Coe et al., 1980; Elias et al., 1980; Smith et al., 1981; National Institute for Occupational Safety and Health, 1981).

Several aspects of the designs of most of these surveys are problematic and limit the inferences that can be drawn from them (see Chapter 2). The comfort and visual performance of VDT workers are important concerns. Unfortunately, however, studies have not established which factors in VDT work--e.g., image quality, lighting conditions, workstation design, visual task requirements, visual status of workers, job design, and psychosocial variables--are correlated with visual complaints, and no conclusions can be drawn as to whether reported symptoms can be attributed to use of VDTs per se, to other variables not unique to VDT work, or to some combination of these factors. The visual complaints of VDT workers described in the field studies appear to us to be qualitatively similar to complaints reported to clinicians by people of all ages and a wide variety of occupations. However, to detect subtle differences, if any, in the character of visual symptoms among groups of workers, clinical examinations rather than field surveys would be required.

Measurements of Visual Status

In addition to questionnaires on physical symptoms, some field surveys have also included routine measurements of the visual status of VDT workers and comparison groups of workers. Dainoff (1980) and Dainoff and coworkers (1981) found no significant differences in visual acuity or in lateral and vertical phoria measured before and after work on two groups of subjects who worked with VDTs for an average of 47 percent and 75 percent of their working time. Dainoff and coworkers reported that no obvious relationship was found between measures of visual status in individual subjects and subjective complaints of ocular discomfort; their analyses, however, are not described. Coe and coworkers (1980) measured visual acuity, astigmatism, near phorias, amblyopia, and color blindness on four groups of VDT workers performing different tasks (input, editing, question-and-answer, creative) and comparison groups of non-VDT workers: no differences between VDT and non-VDT workers were found on any of the measures except for acuity. The non-VDT workers had a higher prevalence of acuity defects, but this difference cannot be interpreted because none of the groups was measured for acuity before workers began their current job. Thus, in contrast to the findings of field surveys regarding visual discomfort and diffi-culties with seeing, defects in visual status have not been reported to occur more frequently among VDT workers than among non-VDT workers (see also the following section and the discussion later in this chapter).

Experimental Field and Laboratory Studies of Visual Functions in VDT Work[1]

Several investigators have attempted to determine whether various visual functions change during performance of VDT tasks; the investigations have covered periods of up to several hours. In some cases, attempts have also been made to compare measures of visual function during VDT and non-VDT tasks. These studies have concluded that transient changes in accommodation (Haider et al., 1980; Östberg, 1980; Östberg et al., 1980; Mourant et al., 1981), convergence (Gunnarsson and Soderberg, 1980), and appar-ent visual acuity (Haider et al., 1980) occur during the use of VDTs. These changes have been asserted to be evidence of "visual fatigue" and have been attributed by the investigators to unusual demands placed on the visual system during video viewing. Two of these studies (Gunnarsson and Soderberg, 1980; Haider et al., 1980) obtained questionnaire data on subjective visual complaints in addition to measuring visual function; however, the relationship between visual complaints and measured changes in visual function apparently was not assessed.

Gunnarsson and Soderberg (1980) measured changes in the near points of accommodation and convergence before, during, and after work in groups of VDT workers under normal and intensified work conditions. They report that some of the subjects showed significant changes in the near point of convergence from the beginning to the end of the workday under the intensified con-dition. The authors concluded that the study shows changes in the

---

[1]These studies are discussed in more detail in Appendix A.

near point of convergence to be a useful objective measure of visual strain associated with VDT work.

Haider and coworkers (1980) measured visual acuity at 4 m in VDT workers performing a test protocol in a work setting and in a comparison group of non-VDT workers performing normal office work (primarily typing). They reported that a temporary reduction in visual acuity occurred following work in the VDT group while the comparison group showed almost no change in acuity. The authors referred to the reduction in acuity as "temporary myopization" resulting from "accommodation strain."

Östberg (1980) and Östberg and coworkers (1980) measured accommodative response and dark focus before and after work in three groups of VDT workers--a group of air traffic controllers and two groups of telephone office VDT workers--each of which performed different types of tasks. Östberg and coworkers reported a shift in dark focus and a reduction in accommodative response in the air traffic controllers and similar but smaller changes in the other two groups. They attributed these results to "visual fatigue" associated with VDT work; the larger changes in the air traffic controllers were attributed to the greater visual demands of their work.

Mourant and coworkers (1981), in a laboratory study, measured the time taken to focus from a near to a far target (referred to as outfocus time) and back to the near target (referred to as infocus time) as a function of the type of visual display used, CRT or hard copy, and time on the task. The authors reported that both outfocus and infocus times were higher for subjects when viewing the CRT and that, for both types of display, times increased as a function of time on task. The authors interpreted these results as evidence of fatigue in the accommodative or eye movement systems, or both. They concluded that use of a CRT has a "measurable fatigue impact on the visual mechanisms" and that this effect is greater for viewing VDTs than for viewing hard copy.

Our analysis of these experimental field and laboratory studies indicates that, because of various aspects in the design, analysis, and interpretation of data, the results cannot be interpreted with any certainty. All of the studies used samples of opportunity; little information was presented on demographic variables and on the working environments of the different groups examined in the studies, despite their possible effects on outcomes. Appropriate control groups were not used; thus it is not possible to attribute the results of the studies specifically to VDT work. While Haider and coworkers used a comparison group, that group did not perform a task comparable to that of the VDT group, and they presented no information on how the two groups compared on other variables. No information was presented in any of the studies on the visual status of the subjects prior to the experiments or on the range of normal variability the subjects might be expected to exhibit; such information is, however, critical to evaluating changes in measures of visual function such as those reported in the studies. The field studies compared groups whose VDT tasks were not comparable; thus it is possible that the effects of task variables were confounded with the effects of the VDT. The techniques used in some studies were subject to such influences as general fatigue and motivation of the subjects. Although all of the studies reported results as statistically significant, little or no information was provided on the statistical analyses performed and the level of significance reached.

Furthermore, the assertion in these studies that the reported temporary changes in measures of visual function are evidence of "visual fatigue" is based on the assumption that changes in these measures of visual function reflect changes in the fatigue state of the oculomotor system; this connection has not been scientifically established, despite an enormous amount of research on the issue over the past 50 years. Workers have been concerned that using VDTs might damage their eyes; however, our analysis (see below) of the temporary changes in measured visual function reported to follow VDT work, as well as non-VDT visual tasks, finds no suggestion of damage (in the sense of long-term irreversible anatomical or physiological changes) to the visual system. However, there does not seem to have been any research specifically to this point.

The Need for Job and Task Analysis

VDTs are used in many occupations, and jobs involving VDT work are highly diverse (see Chapter 1). VDT jobs differ on many dimensions: for example, in the visual tasks involved, the time spent viewing the VDT, the familiarity of the information processed, and the work schedule. These factors shape the visual requirements placed on a worker and presumably affect the likelihood that visual and other complaints will occur. Unfortunately, this diversity has seldom been considered in VDT studies. There has not yet been any well-designed research showing that there are characteristic sources of discomfort unique to VDT work, and the visual tasks characteristic of VDT jobs and non-VDT jobs have not been systematically compared.

Any useful attempt to determine which factors may contribute to visual discomfort should include an analysis of job and task features. Such an analysis would consider how the eyes must be used to perform the task required. For example, in some data entry jobs the worker may only occasionally be required to view the video screen. In such jobs the primary visual task may be reading hard copy from a document holder, a task also performed in many non-VDT jobs. Any visual discomfort experienced in this case would probably not be caused by the VDT itself. In contrast, some VDT jobs require prolonged viewing of the video screen, and many jobs require repetitive eye and head movements between the video screen and hard-copy materials. A systematic research program would be required to determine the relative effects of display characteristics, hard-copy characteristics, and other workstation features on the comfort and performance of workers in particular jobs.

Psychosocial factors also may affect the experiencing and reporting of symptoms of visual discomfort. Workers in some jobs are allowed sufficient flexibility to temporarily modify their work pattern if they experience visual discomfort. Other jobs, however, are much more rigid in time and activity requirements. It also seems likely that job satisfaction will affect workers' tolerance for discomfort and their reporting of symptoms.

The quality of VDT workstation design varies greatly even within given job categories. Worker comfort and performance can be affected substantially by display quality (Chapter 4), lighting and reflections (Chapter 5), and anthropometric features (Chapter 6). Thus, job analyses should include consideration of the quality of these factors in individual workstations. Some problems with workstation features and visual task requirements are clearly not unique to VDT jobs: for example, workers in various non-VDT jobs—secretaries, editors, teachers, etc.--must read hard copy or handwriting of poor legibility. In some VDT jobs, workers must deal with both poor-quality video displays and poor-quality hard copy, and they may experience cumulative effects in task difficulty and the effort required.

Are There Unique Features of VDT Tasks?

Textual characters generated by VDTs differ in several respects from hard-copy characters. The effects of some of these display parameters on reading performance are discussed in Chapter 4. The self-luminous nature of a VDT and the transient presentation of material are obvious differences. Noticeable differences may also occur in contrast, sharpness of characters, image stability, and other features. Murch (1982a) argues, on the basis of a comparison of accommodative response to CRTs and hard copy, that CRT displays generally do not provide a visual stimulus capable of evoking optimal accommodation; the data he reports, however, do not seem to support this conclusion.[2]

VDTs typically use simplified fonts, chosen for engineering convenience, that contrast with the hard-copy fonts that have evolved through applied research and many years of practical experience. Image quality of a given display will in part determine how well it compares to hard copy in terms of worker performance and comfort, but the quality (especially legibility) of hard copy is not always good either, especially in cases of photocopies, carbons, and computer printouts.

Problems with lighting and reflections are, of course, encountered in reading hard copy as well as in viewing VDTs, but some aspects of VDTs can be particularly problematic. For example, it is possible that users' accommodation and convergence may fluctuate between the characters displayed on the screen and images reflected on the screen (which are at a different optical distance), and this may adversely affect comfort and performance (see Chapter 5). VDT workstation design can also present difficulties similar to but more pronounced than those encountered in traditional clerical workstations. For example, VDT workstations may impose additional postural constraints and requirements for head and eye movements (see Chapter 6).

Both visual and nonvisual aspects of VDT work are shaped by the character of the person-computer interaction. Business forms and text have evolved through centuries of use, while VDT formats have been designed primarily in accordance with programmers' notions as to what will be efficient or convenient to the user. Research on VDT format design and its effects has barely begun (Granda, 1980; Kolers et al., 1981). It is important to note that the software of a computer program sets the stage and determines the rules for interaction. Employees who function as lower-level users of a computer system play an especially sub-

---

[2]Murch used a laser optometer to measure the immediate accommodative responses of subjects to a pattern of X's displayed at a distance of 50 cm on six types of VDTs and on negative contrast hard copy. The accommodative response to each display varied only slightly from the ideal value of 2.0 diopters, ranging from 1.84 to 2.14 (the value for hard copy was 2.01), and all fell within the expected 0.25-diopter depth of field expected under the measurement conditions of the study. No statistical analyses are reported, but the differences in measured refractive status do not appear to be significant. It is arguable whether the underlying premise of this study, that the accuracy of focus in response to a display provides an index of visibility for that display, is reasonable.

servient role to its programming--a role that requires them to place strong dependence on the entire computer system to carry out their jobs. There is, however, growing interest in designing "user-friendly" computer systems (see, e.g., Association for Computing Machinery et al., 1982).

In contrast to hard copy, VDT text is often active and transient in nature. For example, text may be <u>scrolled</u>, moved up the screen to expose new material at the bottom and cover up preceding material at the top. The few studies of scrolling undertaken to date (e.g., Kolers et al., 1981; Sekey and Teitz, 1982) do not suggest a problem. Kolers and coworkers found little difference in observed eye movements between reading a static display and scrolled text, especially when the scrolled display was rapidly paced. The effect of scrolling on worker comfort over prolonged periods, however, has not been examined.

Adequate research that would establish whether there is anything inherent in VDT tasks that can unavoidably cause visual difficulties not encountered in comparable non-VDT tasks has not been conducted. We suggest, however, that attention to quality of display design, control of lighting and reflections, and appropriate job design (including display format and structure of operator-VDT interaction) would go a long way toward preventing difficulties (see Chapter 9). Research on the effects of VDT work on the visual comfort and performance of workers should be designed to distinguish which factors (e.g., observable jitter, flicker, screen-reflected images, poor design and format) contribute to which effects and whether problems can be reduced by changing display parameters. Without such research, development of effective displays and comfortable interaction conventions will depend on the slow and uncertain processes of evolution by trial and error.

The Special Task of Reading

Reading is a central task in most VDT and comparable non-VDT jobs. Display characteristics that affect short-term reading performance are discussed in Chapter 4. There has been little research systematically comparing sustained reading (for several hours) from VDTs and from printed materials. Bagnara (1980) found a decrease in performance in an error-detecting task over two hours of reading short news articles from VDTs, but the study failed to counterbalance the materials, it used only six operators, and--most important for the present point--it did not separate effects due to the reading task per se from those due to the VDT per se. Several studies have reported temporary changes in oculomotor function that were argued to result specifically from

VDT work; the findings of these studies are critically examined later in this chapter and in Appendix A.

If significant oculomotor changes, decrements in reading performance, or visual discomfort were specific to VDT work (which has not been established), one would want to know what aspects of reading were affected by VDT characteristics. Appropriately designed research is needed to compare the effects of different kinds of reading tasks on the visual-motor system and to examine the interaction of those effects with specific characteristics of VDTs. (The aspects of the reading task that would need to be considered are discussed below, and the relevant video display characteristics are discussed in Chapter 9.)

The reading task requires a viewer to discriminate some or all of the symbols or strings of symbols from others of the set of symbols that might have been presented (for example, to distinguish the letter $\underline{A}$ from other letters of the alphabet). This discrimination task requires that a reader's eyes maintain some minimum degree of focus or accommodation and be directed so that the part of the array about which information is needed projects to the fovea of the eye. Visual acuity falls off very rapidly outside the fovea: only about four individual letters can be read as such without moving the eye, although characteristic word forms and lengths can, when they constitute meaningful text, convey some information for considerably longer distances from the fovea (up to 12 letter spaces) (see Woodworth, 1938; McConkie and Rayner, 1975, 1976). Muscular activity is therefore needed to maintain accommodation and to move the eye to new fixations (through eye movements called saccades, discussed below). The fineness of detail that must be resolved varies greatly with the nature of the display itself and with the task. With dense and nonredundant text, a reader may need to resolve every distinctive feature of each symbol, while with highly redundant or familiar material, much less detail is needed to perform the same task. One reading task (e.g., proofreading) may require much more detailed vision than another (e.g., skimming for gist). The precision of accommodation and the number of saccades that are needed to perform any task with any given body of text depend on the legibility of the display, the meaningful structure of the text, the nature of the reading task, and the reader's skills.

The effects on reading performance of such variables as font, letter and word spacing, letter size, organization of materials on a page, contrast between letter and background, and reflectance or texture of the paper have been studied to some degree. The largest effects under normal circumstances are associated with the content of the material and its relation to the cognitive task, i.e., the variables of cognitive organization (Breland and Breland,

1944; Paterson and Tinker, 1956; Tinker, 1965; Bouma, 1980; Engel, 1980; Timmers et al., 1980; Treurniet, 1980).

According to this conception of reading, tasks that involve low levels of cognitive demand allow a great deal of visual imperfection: a lot of redundant information in a text allows a reader to miss a great deal and still "see" everything needed for the task. For more difficult reading tasks, a viewer is forced to process at the word-by-word or letter-by-letter level, and there is a greater cognitive load. Such a lack of redundancy places great demands on attention, which in turn requires both sustained concentration and detailed vision. The tasks that might create such cognitive load when performed under pressures for speed and accuracy include data entry or acquisition of nonredundant and unfamiliar materials. Such tasks would place more stringent demands on the discrimination of detail throughout the text. Although the rate of saccades does not appear to change much with task difficulty (Judd and Buswell, 1922), the saccades must be smaller and more precisely placed so that the fixations are closer together, and the emphasis on discriminating individual letters may place more stringent demands on the accommodative mechanisms.

The Problematic Concepts of "Visual Fatigue" and "Eyestrain"

The literature on visual complaints and symptoms of VDT workers contains many references to "visual fatigue" and "eyestrain," but these terms are often ambiguous.

Carmichael and Dearborn, in their classic treatise Reading and Visual Fatigue (1947), discuss the topic in the context of problems encountered in research on fatigue in general. They consider fatigue to have three aspects: the subjective experience of an individual performing prolonged work; changes in task performance over time; and physiological changes. In studies of these three aspects, there has been little success in relating changes in physiological parameters observed in fatigue experiments to either task performance or subjective aspects (Cameron, 1973; Smith, 1979).

The Carmichael and Dearborn study illustrates many of the issues encountered in research on effects of prolonged performance of visual tasks. They found no decrement in reading comprehension or eye movement performance (number of fixations and regressions) over a six-hour period among high school and college subjects reading hard-copy or microfilm text. Many of the subjects reported increasing tiredness or general discomfort over the six-hour period, but it appeared to be related more to the constraints on posture and activity than to the visual task. Apparently there were only a few ocular or visual complaints (the subjects were not questioned specifically about visual or ocular symptoms but were asked to describe their subjective responses in general).

The results of the Carmichael and Dearborn study contrast with the finding by Hoffman (1946) of decrements in reading performance by students over a four-hour period. Carmichael and Dearborn attributed the difference to motivation. Their study, unlike Hoffman's, employed incentives to maintain a high level of reading performance. Some studies have reported that highly motivated subjects can maintain effective task performance (e.g., driving or flying) for many hours even though they experience symptoms of subjective fatigue (e.g., tiredness, discomfort, sleepiness, reluctance to continue work), while other studies have reported decreased performance of tasks in periods as short as two hours (see Cameron, 1973). The discrepancies among these studies may be a function of the increasing effort required to maintain performance over time, the level of arousal evoked by the particular tasks, and the motivation of the subjects.

According to Duke-Elder and Abrams (1970:559), "Eyestrain may be defined as the symptoms experienced in the conscious striving of the visual apparatus to clarify vision by ineffectual adjustments" (see also Borish, 1970). Other authors (e.g., Ferguson et al., 1974) have objected to the term "eyestrain," which might suggest damage to the eyes. Asthenopia (used in general to refer to any subjective visual symptoms or distress resulting from use of one's eyes) may be a more useful term. Duke-Elder and Abrams classify the symptoms, which are quite varied, as visual (especially blurring), ocular (the eyes feel tired, hot, uncomfortable, or painful), referral (e.g., headaches), and functional (behavioral). The ocular discomfort is said to be due to muscular fatigue, but the mechanisms are not known. Duke-Elder and Abrams emphasize the role of higher perceptual processes in tiring from continuous effort to interpret blurred and indistinct images. The causes of asthenopia are described as environmental (involving illumination, the nature of visual tasks, and the characteristics of the objects viewed), ocular (the patient's visual status), and constitutional (involving both physical health and emotional state).

Refractive Errors and Visual Difficulties

There are a number of clinical conditions involving small uncorrected refractive errors and oculomotor imbalances that can cause visual difficulties with prolonged near work or critical detail work. When a person attempts to rectify those refractive errors or imbalances by continuous muscular effort, symptoms of asthenopia can develop. Such symptoms can be caused by uncorrected ametropia, accommodative difficulties (see also the next section), heterophoria, convergence difficulties, fusional inadequacy, or aniseikonia. It is possible that some of the visual complaints of some VDT workers (as well as those of non-VDT workers) might involve such clincial conditions. In such cases, a careful clinical examination would be useful, and refraction may relieve the symptoms.

Myopia

Myopia (nearsightedness) is an extremely common abnormality of ocular refraction occurring in varying degrees in almost one-quarter of the adult population of the United States (Roberts, 1978). Myopia is less common in populations that are less technologically advanced (Taylor, 1981), and it is more common and of greater degree in adults than in children (Sorsby, 1972). For these reasons it has been suggested that excessive use of the eyes for near work is the cause of myopia. There is, however, considerable controversy about the interaction of near work and myopia (Bear and Richler, 1982; Taylor, 1982). As we discussed above, it is not clear whether the characteristics of VDTs or of the visual tasks performed in working with them differ from characteristics of other forms of near work with regard to a possible interaction with ocular refraction.

OCULOMOTOR FACTORS
AFFECTING VISUAL PERFORMANCE

As discussed above, the concept of visual fatigue is one that has escaped canonical scientific definition, and there has been little progress in relating subjective measures of fatigue to performance of visual tasks or physiological functions. Several investigators have measured oculomotor functions during prolonged performance of visual tasks (including VDT work) with the hope of finding objective correlates of visual complaints or even a phsyiological basis for those complaints. Recently, some investigators have argued that temporary changes in oculomotor functions reported to follow VDT work are evidence of visual fatigue. This argument is problematic for several reasons (some of which were discussed above): the decrement in motor performance response to a stimulus may be due to adaptation of the sensory organs, habituation of central nervous system activity, or decline in motivation, as well as to true muscular fatigue. The effects of subjective (general) fatigue may in some cases be reversed by increased motivation. Efficiency, the ratio of response to effort, has been suggested to be a more appropriate measure of fatigue than response decrement, but of course, efficiency--like subjective fatigue--is difficult to measure (Cameron, 1973). Furthermore, observed oculomotor changes might in some cases be normal adaptive responses to sustained work rather than indications of declining performance.

In this section we discuss oculomotor factors that have been studied during sustained performance of visual tasks. The general functions of the oculomotor system are described to provide a context for considering the temporary changes that have been reported to follow sustained visual performance. We discuss the difficulties in relating these reported oculomotor changes to complaints of visual discomfort, and we review studies that have used visual tasks such as reading printed materials and microfilm, inspection tasks, tracking tasks, and, more recently, reading from VDTs.

Eye Movements

Eye-movement changes during sustained performance of visual tasks may be considered at several different levels of extraoculomotor function: saccadic trajectory, dual-mode tracking movements, higher-level eye movements, and gaze and the vestibulo-ocular reflex.

Saccadic Trajectory

The eye (specifically, the fovea, the high-resolution, color-sensitive portion of the retina) is directed rapidly from one object of regard to another by saccadic movements. The performance of saccades has been examined in considerable detail, anatomic (Carpenter, 1977; Graybiel, 1977; Keller, 1977), physiologic (Bach-y-Rita, 1971; Evinger et al., 1977), and control-system theoretic (Stark, 1968, 1971; Robinson, 1981). A change of fixation of the eye involving a saccade is caused by a burst of neural activity to the extraocular agonist muscles. The activity rises to a peak value and then settles back to a lower plateau (Robinson, 1964; Fuchs and Luschei, 1970; Collins, 1975), a pattern sometimes called a pulse-step. Hering's law of equal innervation requires that the same pulse-step be applied to the corresponding muscles of both eyes.

In normal circumstances the trajectories of saccades are stereotypical, and if certain parameters of the saccades (e.g., peak acceleration and peak velocity) are plotted against each other, a smooth curve called the main sequence is obtained.

Surprisingly, at least in adults, there is remarkably little variation in the main sequence (Bogen et al., 1974; Able et al., 1979), and it can therefore be used as a yardstick to measure changes in performance. The fine neurological control structure of the saccadic trajectory has been shown to decompose rapidly (within minutes) in repetitive tracking[3] situations in at least two very different ways. First, central nervous system habituation allows the appearance of double saccades, each component of which falls naturally on the main sequence (Bahill and Stark, 1975). The fact that these fit the main sequence provides evidence that even lower-level pulse-shaping neurons in the brainstem (as well as, of course, neuromuscular and muscular factors) are functioning quite normally. Thus, it is clear in this instance at least that a well-documented appearance of oculomotor fatigue has been definitely localized to the central nervous system. This is especially important because increased motivational effort is known to compensate for fatigue processes; thus, it is often logically difficult to prove that the fatigue process does not lie in the peripheral neuromuscular apparatus (as one might expect). Also, pulse-step mismatches in the controller signal envelopes of neuronal bursting and tonic firing of nerve impulses occur and result in "glissades," which often violate Hering's law of equal innervation to corresponding muscles (Bahill and Stark, 1975; Bahill et al., 1976).

Second, the more peripheral neuromuscular fatigue type of decomposition of the saccadic trajectory produces generally slowed movements below the main sequence velocity-amplitude relationship and also irregular fragments showing erratic profiles of velocity and acceleration. These fragments have been found in patients with peripheral neural and neuromuscular diseases (Feldon et al., 1982) and lie above the main sequence as a result of "truncation" (similar to the truncation that occurs in overlapping voluntary nystagmus saccades) (Stark et al., 1980).

---

[3]Reading VDT displays is largely performed by repetitive saccades at a rate of approximately four saccades per second. Thus there are similarities and differences between reading eye movements and repetitive tracking eye movements. Students of reading eye movements use tracking movements as a related but simpler form of sequential reading eye movements. Indeed, Pavlides (1981) has suggested that a deficiency in tracking accompanies abnormalities in reading eye movements (see discussion of reading eye movements above).

Dual Mode Tracking Eye Movements

A second level of eye movement performance has to do with both smooth pursuit and saccadic eye movements. In the continual activity of moving one's eyes, an interactive dual-mode control system acts to turn the eyes conjugately (binocularly) throughout the visual field. In order to study these spontaneous movements, physiologists and bioengineers have developed a tracking task[4]--very similar to a test of skill in a penny arcade, where one tries to aim at a moving target—in which the task is to aim the eyes quickly and accurately. In this test a single entire saccadic response may drop out, and the sequence of responses then continues in phase with an alternating jumping target (Lion and Brockhurst, 1951). In addition, the tracking quality itself may deteriorate with gradually increased reaction times (minutes) and abnormal sequences of saccades (Stark et al., 1962). Saccadic smooth pursuit may also occur as a compensatory adaptation when the gain of smooth pursuit decreases.[5] Visual feedback is a crucial element in the control of eye movements at this level.

Higher-Level Eye Movement Patterns

Reading A third level of eye movement performance comprises reading and looking, which are composed of sequential patterns of saccadic eye movements. The reading task is complex, with cognitive, linguistic, visual, and eye movement factors all interacting (Huey, 1908 [1968]; Woodworth, 1938; Hochberg, 1970; Smith, 1971; Fisher, 1975; McConkie and Rayner, 1975; Just and Carpenter, 1978; Rayner, 1978; Scinto, 1978; Stern, 1978; O'Regan, 1979;

---

[4] The tracking task is an excellent paradigm for human factors experimentation to define operator activities, for example, in controlling vehicles. In regard to the eye movement control system, the tracking task has been studied with the conceptual and mathematical tools of the control engineer (Fender and Nye, 1961; Young and Stark, 1963). So far this methodology has not been applied to VDT use, but it is a very powerful tool for the quantitative study of task performance and its deterioration with sustained activity. Future studies of fatigue with VDT use would benefit from application of this methodology. It is important to note again Cameron's notion of efficiency: effort may compensate for decreased response and may maintain performance in highly motivated subjects (Cameron, 1973).
[5] Restoration may occur after a brief rest period (tens of seconds) or a startle dishabituation stimulus.

Spiro et al., 1980). Many studies have demonstrated poorer reading performance with less-than-optimal typography or illumination (Tinker, 1939; Tinker and Paterson, 1939; Demilia, 1968). However, several experienced and careful researchers have found no significant decrement in reading performance after six hours of reading concentrated material (Carmichael and Dearborn, 1947; Carmichael, 1951-1952).[6] The eye-movement component of the reading task involves mainly a sequential pattern of saccades, about one for each word, although small common words (a, of, the) are often skipped.[7] About 10 to 20 percent of the saccades are regressions or backward saccades, generally to a linguistically critical word in the syntax of the sentence. Indeed, the French word verification for a regression assumes this linguistic role. At the end of a line, a larger saccade sweeps the eye to the left margin of the next line, and numerous corrective saccades occur, especially vertical saccades to place the eyes correctly on the line. Large saccades, such as occur when a user looks from a dark VDT to illuminated hard copy, may provide a light stimulus to the pupil and may also quickly change focal distance and stimulate an accommodative response. Vergence and accommodative response have not been thoroughly studied during reading.

[6]Although Carmichael and Dearborn (1947) reported that subjects who had spent several hours reading such concentrated material as Adam Smith's Wealth of Nations reported feeling fatigued, 60 of the 80 subjects felt they could continue to read if provided a rest. [7]Reading rates of 300 words per minute are near maximum. The maximum rate of saccadic generation is 5 per second, which is equivalent to a reading rate of 300 words per minute (Adler-Grinberg and Stark, 1978). (The extra number of regression saccades is roughly equated to the number of skipped small words.) This high frequency of saccades must be considered as a possible source of interaction with the flicker produced by VDT regeneration rates (David Bridgeman, Department of Psychology, University of California, Santa Cruz, personal communication, 1981).

Many studies have shown that poor readers with or without specific dyslexia often have irregular reading eye movement patterns and prolonged fixations. These and backward staircases have been found in peripheral motor dyslexia secondary to the diplopia of a peripheral oculomotor paresis. One may speculate that minor forms of dyslexia in VDT operators may surface and produce complaints.

Picture Scanning Some VDT users examine graphs or charts, and engineers engaged in computer-assisted design (CAD) typically work with orthographic projections or perspective displays of machine components. It is possible that some of these workers examine diagrams with sequences of eye movements that have been dubbed scanpaths. The scanpath, which is observed under certain laboratory conditions, is a nonrandom sequence of saccadic eye movements that scans a picture in an idiosyncratic pattern for each subject. Scanpaths appear to be generated by internal cognitive models in a checking phase of pattern recognition. Recent evidence for this comes from the work of Stark, Noton, and Ellis who used ambiguous and fragmented figures and asked subjects to signal their alternating perceptions (Noton and Stark, 1971a, 1971b, 1971c; Stark and Ellis, 1981). With the same subject and the same physical pictures, the eye-movement scanpath developed different patterns, each associated with a particular perception. Scanpaths are modified with continued examination of the same pattern (Yarbus, 1967), but the implications of this finding are not known. Minor changes in scanpaths may not be noticed.[8]

Gaze and the Vestibulo-Ocular Reflex

The vestibulo-ocular reflex is a primitive phylogenetic mechanism that stabilizes the direction of gaze in space. In the brainstem there are connections between the oculomotor system and the vestibular apparatus that monitor balance and posture with respect to gravity. If a head movement occurs, a signal that generates a compensatory eye movement (in the absence of volition) is sent from the vestibular apparatus to the oculomotor system. Thus, when looking at a visual target, a person may turn his or her body or head without losing visual contact (Baloh and Honrubia, 1979; Wilson and Jones, 1979; Henn et al., 1980).

Coordinated gaze movement normally has an initial eye-in-orbit saccade onto the target followed by a synkinetic and much slower head movement. At the level of the electromyographic (EMG) signal, latencies are synchronous, but because the visco-

---

[8]Drivers engaged in long, continuing driving tasks show central concentrations of eye fixations rather than normal, widespread, active looking and searching patterns (McDowell and Rockwell, 1978). The question of preview control, how far ahead the driver looks, may be important to the concentration of fixations by fatigue (Tomizuka and Whitney, 1975).

inertial dynamics of head and neck muscles are different from the viscoelastic dynamics of eye and extraocular muscles, the saccade is over before the head position has changed. The vestibulo-ocular reflex generated by head acceleration drives the compensatory eye movement, eye-in-orbit, in the opposite direction so that gaze, eye-in-space, remains on target. Thus, gaze movement has the advantage of the rapidity of the eye saccade, and at the end of the movement the eye is in primary position in the orbit and the target is in the straightforward position, since directional sense is determined by head position.

Diseases of the oculomotor system, the vestibular apparatus, or the central nervous system may cause incomplete visual compensation for body movement. In such circumstances a disequilibrium may result because visual space does not correspond with the subject's egocentric image of space. This sensation results in nausea, vomiting, and vertigo. The same symptoms may occur in the absence of disease if a person uses psychotropic drugs such as tranquilizers, sedatives, or alcohol (Rashbass and Russel, 1961; Wilkinson et al., 1974; Barmack and Pettorosi, 1980; Favilla et al., 1981).

Blinking

There are two forms of blinking motion, a reflex action occurring about once in every 2 to 10 seconds, and voluntary-force eye closure (Hung et al., 1977). Blinking stimulates tear production and provides a pumping-out action for contaminants in the eye.[9] The normal blink rate decreases with age and with the use of drugs such as tranquilizers. An abnormally high or low rate of blinking may be related (although no clinical evidence exists) to the ocular irritation syndrome of redness and injection (i.e., hyperemia) of sclera and cornea, the sensation of heat and burning of the anterior portion of the eye, and headache.

Some visual tasks requiring concentrated attention reduce the rate of blinking (which may lead to dry eyes and irritation), but excessive blinking has been associated with reading difficult text.

----

[9]Transient quenching of the light input to the rods and cones of the retina may have a resetting effect on the excitability of these receptors and all of the subsequent visual neurons--that is, the bipolar, horizontal, amacrine, and ganglion cells of the retina and neurons in the lateral geniculate body; the visual cortex; the parietal cortex; and the frontal eye fields. Thus blinking could be considered both as a corneal and as a visual "windshield wiper."

Blinking has been reported to be associated with fatigue since at least 1895 (Katz, as reported by Kravklov, 1974; Bartley, 1942; Luckiesh, 1947; Krivohlavy et al., 1969), but it has also been denied (Bitterman, 1945, 1946, 1947; Brozek et al., 1950; Wood et al., 1950; Holland and Tarlow, 1972).

Luckiesh and Moss (1937, 1942) conducted a number of experiments and concluded that the rate of involuntary blinking was a dependable criterion for ease of seeing. Subsequent work by McFarland and coworkers (1942), Bitterman (1945, 1946), and Tinker (1946), which failed to support Luckiesh's findings, touched off a debate in the literature (Bitterman, 1946, 1947; Luckiesh, 1946, 1947). Luckiesh defended his results, claiming that the different experimental conditions used by other investigators naturally led to different results. Bitterman and others argued that any measure that required strict and rather narrow conditions could not be used as an index of "visual effort" or "visual fatigue."

A later study by Tinker attempted to repeat in as much detail as possible the conditions of the Luckiesh and Moss experiments. Tinker was unable to confirm their results and concludes (Tinker, 1949:560): "Under the conditions of this experiment, rate of involuntary blinking does not reflect differences in ease of seeing." Brozek and coworkers (1950) measured several ocular functions at different time intervals for subjects performing "hard visual work" and found no significant increase in the blink rate. Finally, Wood and Bitterman (1950) had subjects perform a reading task in which visual effort and performance were varied separately. They found that blink rate was independent of visual effort but was inversely correlated with performance.

Triadic Near Reflex: Combined Focusing, Convergence, and Aperture Mechanisms

The mechanisms of the near reflex, that is, the triad of vergence, accommodation, and pupil diameter, are closely interlinked, each exerting some control on the other. This section first considers each mechanism separately and then discusses interactions between the three.

Accommodation

Focusing is achieved by both a lentincular and an extralenticular mechanism. The active ciliary muscle applies tension and stretches the peripheral portion of the zonule of Zinn, which causes the lenticular portion of the system to assume a particular shape (i.e., a particular state of accommodation) determined by the elasticity of the lens and surrounding capsule.[10]

Blur is one of the stimuli for accommodation (Fincham, 1937, 1951; Allen, 1955; Phillips and Stark, 1977) and is detected via the foveal cones under photopic light conditions. While blur can tell the accommodative control system that the image is out of focus, a static value of blur is an even error signal: that is, it cannot indicate which way to change the accommodation in order to correct the error. The system overcomes this deficit by acting as a hill-climbing controller.[11] In this way the control system can determine the direction of change that reduces blur and can then initiate a steady change in that direction until blur is minimized.

The question of blur introduces a possible factor in visual distress during use of VDTs. The inexpensive terminals in use in many VDT installations have some inherent design features that prevent them from producing sharply defined (i.e., resolvable or legible) characters (Sakrison, 1977; Kajiya and Ullner, 1981). The accommodative mechanism of a user's eye might therefore be robbed of the error signal it needs in order to achieve good visual acuity. This may also affect the comfort of VDT operators. Many other clues help the accommodative mechanism. Through synkinesis, for example, the vergence mechanism can produce a change in accommodation without requiring a blur signal to drive accommodation directly (see above).

The accommodative system has a control-bias level with a set point of about 1 diopter (although there is considerable variation among people in this value). Accommodation drifts to this bias

---

[10]Thus the dual, indirect, active theory of the accommodative mechanism was put forward by Helmholtz (1867) and has received support over the past century (Rohen and Rentsch, 1969; Saladin and Stark, 1975). It is a dual mechanism because both lenticular and extralenticular elements participate, indirect because the ciliary muscle does not act directly on the lens as a sphincter but acts indirectly by unloading the axial portion of the ciliary ligament, and active because activity in the ciliary muscle produces an increase in accommodation.

[11]See Stark (1968) for a discussion of the concept of a hill-climbing controller (which attempts to minimize blur but does not try to correct to zero error). The accommodative mechanism also has many other nonlinear characteristics (Stark, 1968). It also has a leaky integrator (Krishnan and Stark, 1975) or leaky memory with about a 10-second time constant.

level[12] by reducing illumination below photopic levels (night myopia), by removing a focusable image (space myopia) (Whiteside, 1957), or by making the system "open loop" by electronic methods (Phillips and Stark, 1977). The accommodative control-bias level is sometimes called the dark focus. It is not peculiar to darkness, however; it applies equally to empty-field conditions and to open-loop conditions. Because the bias level is set by synkinetic control of the vergence system (see above), it is not a true focused state of accommodation.

Static Factors in Accommodation   The range of accommodation is up to 16 diopters in children but only about 10 diopters in young adults. The gradual restriction of range of accommodation is called presbyopia, but since it begins in childhood, it is clearly not a degenerative condition.[13] By the age of 40, normal adults need reading glasses or bifocals as a static refractive prosthesis.[14] Certain other static disabilities are seen clinically. Accommodative spasm (fixed accommodation at the near point) usually also involves vergence, indicating that it originates in abnormal central nervous system control rather than in ocular muscles. Accommodative asthenopia (fixed accommodation at the far point) occurs without evident accommodative effort, again suggesting that the ciliary muscles are not involved. Because these static conditions occur most frequently in persons aged 30-40 years, they may be related to the development of presbyopia. Accommodative spasm and accommodative asthenopia are examples of minor ocular deficits that may be related to the incidence of complaints of ocular discomfort in VDT users.

---

[12]The drift toward bias level is called a lead by clinicians when the subject is focusing at infinity and a lazy lag when the subject is focusing at a near target.

[13]The ciliary muscle has normal strength and activity (Saladin and Stark, 1975), but since the growth of the lens continues, producing a larger lens with a decreased curvature and increased radius, there is a recession of the near point.

[14]Meredith Morgan, Elwin Marg, and Lawrence W. Stark believe that by the time one understands the mechanisms of accommodation, pupillary contraction is one's only mechanism of accommodation; that is, increasing the depth of focus by pupillary constriction is the only way in which a presbyope can approach his or her near point.

Dynamic Factors in Accommodation The latency of accommodation and the rate at which it can be changed vary among subjects and for the same subject under different conditions (Shirachi et al., 1978).[15] Disfacility of accommodation, which is less severe than accommodative spasm or accommodative asthenopia, shows responses delayed beyond the usual latency and slowed rates of change (Liu et al., 1979).[16] Responses reach the required accommodative levels but then drift back. Oscillation in level of accommodation beyond that normally found in healthy subjects can also occur.

Fatigue and Accommodation

The earliest work on fatigue and accommodation consisted of clinical impressions only, and there continues to be clinical literature (e.g., Weber, 1950). Ergographic studies have been performed for the last 50 years (Lancaster and Williams, 1914; Howe, 1916; Blatt, 1931; Berens and Stark, 1932; Kurtz, 1937, 1938; Hofstetter, 1943; Ostberg, 1980; and Kintz and Bowker, 1982).[17] Some of these studies have found deficits in accommodation that

---

[15]Methods of experimentally and clinically analyzing these dynamics include ergographic recordings and, more recently, the laser optometer. In these methods the subject positions the target so that it falls within his or her depth of focus. This positioning may be recorded as a measure of subjective appreciation of blur or laser speckle direction. A new laser ergograph method depends upon subjective appreciation of directional movement of a "speckle pattern" secondary to separation of the conjugate plane of the image from the retina. The image is formed by a rotating drum illuminated by a laser. Objective methods of analyzing accommodative dynamics include: the lensometer principle, which measures the blur of a target on the retina; the Scheiner method, in which blur is converted to prismatic shift (Malmstrom et al., 1981); retinoscopic methods, which use directional image motion as an indication of accommodation error; and the third Purkinje image method (O'Neill and Stark, 1968), which directly measures lens anterior pole position.

[16]It is interesting that both presbyopes and children can show accommodative disfacility. Both subjective (Hofstetter, 1943) and objective (Liu et al., 1979) observations have shown that disfacility can be successfully treated by exercise.

[17]The ergograph was designed to measure and record objectively a sequence of continual movements so that if fatigue occurs and the amplitude of the movements decreases, it can be noted.

are usually recessions of the near point during sustained performance of a variety of near-work tasks. They all agree that the results are variable. For example, Gunnarsson and Soderberg (1980) report recessions of the near point for younger VDT workers and some transient approach of the near point during the early part of the day for older VDT workers. Saito and coworkers (1981), however, report approach of the near point with younger workers. Hofstetter feels the rapid restoration with attention indicates that the locus of fatigue is in the central nervous system and not in the muscles; that fatigue shows up in a masked, nonseeing eye almost to the same extent as in a seeing eye (Berens and Sells, 1954) rules out fatigue in sensory processes. Various investigators believe that what is lacking in their research is a distinction between fatigue and boredom and, especially, control of motivational factors that might combat performance decrements. Another basic issue is the question of whether the objective measurements define abnormally functioning accommodation or simply an adaptive response (especially if the pupil becomes smaller). That is, for an overlearned task involving muscular effort, an unconscious response is to reduce muscular effort to the lowest level compatible with task performance. Indeed, most often acuity and other measures of vision remain normal. Perhaps a skilled VDT operator shows an adaptive response that should not be construed as a sign of fatigue.

A few authors have performed dynamic studies with fatigued subjects.[18] Malmstrom and coworkers (1981) used a tracking task in which subjects followed near and far sinusoidally moving targets for a 6.5-minute period. Minor reductions in accommodative amplitude occurred. Logical defects in this study (and in many other studies) include the absence of necessity to maintain sharp focus on the target and the lack of control of possible pupillary constriction. Krivohlavy and coworkers (1969) used subjective methods to show that the rate of change of accommodation was slowed in fatigued subjects, who took longer to cycle fixation between near and far targets; this effect was significantly correlated with reduced performance in a reading task.

Several studies have reported changes in users' accommodation in the course of work at VDTs. These studies have numerous methodological problems that make their interpretation difficult (see the discussion in Appendix A). For example, the study by Gunnarsson and Soderberg (1980) of changes in near points of accommodation and convergence did not include a control group of non-VDT workers performing similar visual tasks. Östberg

---

[18]Krueger (1980) has reviewed the physiology of and the clinical approach to accommodation.

(1980) and Östberg and coworkers (1980) reported decreases in accommodative response and shifts in dark focus point among air traffic controllers after two hours of VDT work. No significant changes were found among two groups of telephone operators performing work involving VDTs. This study did not include any control groups of workers performing similar tasks without VDTs. The authors suggest that the differences in effects among the groups were due to the greater visual demands of air traffic controllers, and they argue that these findings are evidence of "visual fatigue" caused by VDT work. However, the failure to include appropriate control groups, especially in light of the stressful nature of air traffic control work, makes it impossible to determine whether these effects were associated with VDT work per se. Murch (1982b) found no change in dark focus (i.e., bias level), accommodation, or convergence following a two-hour intensive visual search task at either a raster video display or a direct-view storage tube terminal.

Haider and coworkers (1980) reported a very small transient decrease in visual acuity during the course of three hours of VDT work. No change in acuity was found in a non-VDT comparison group performing general office work. However, the work of the comparison group apparently differed from that of the VDT group in several respects, so it cannot be determined whether the reported change in acuity was related specifically to VDT task features. Small differences in acuity were reported between groups that worked with VDTs with green characters and those with yellow characters. Haider and coworkers suggested that the change in acuity signified "temporary myopization," probably due to "accommodation strain." Murch (1982b) also reported a reduction in acuity following visual search at a raster video display, but not with a direct-view storage tube display. The finding suggests that the acuity change was related in some way to the raster display since the two tasks were well matched for other features. Follow-up of this preliminary study would be useful.

Mourant and coworkers (1981) reported that the time required to move eye fixation and focus between near and far points slowed following a visual search task with a video display but not with a hard-copy display. The approach of this study is potentially valuable, but a number of methodological flaws make the results difficult to interpret. Eye movement records were evaluated subjectively, and reliability was not assessed (see Appendix A). Accommodation was probably not a factor in the reported effects since presbyopes and young workers showed similar changes, and both the distances used, 0.16 diopters and (apparently) about 2.2 diopters could have been within the depth of focus of the subjects' eyes at the same time. Murch (1982b) reported that no significant change in focus speed from a near to a far target occurred following VDT work, but he did not include details of his measurement procedures.

In summary, none of the studies reporting oculomotor changes following VDT work has demonstrated that the changes are related to visual task features specific to VDT work. The significance of the reported oculomotor changes is not clear, but no evidence has been presented that they are problematic for workers. A serious defect in these VDT studies, and in other studies described in this section, is that pupillary aperture was not measured. The pupil is known to constrict with sleepiness, boredom, or fatigue and, if constricted, would increase the depth of focus, reducing the requirement for accommodation. Note that unless pupil size is measured and depth of focus calculated, it is not possible to state that a certain measured accommodative state is or is not optimal.

Vergence

Vergence is the oculomotor control system that maintains binocular fixation. As an object moves closer or farther away, the two visual axes rotate disjunctively and symmetrically to maintain bifixation on the point of interest. Vergence uses the same muscles as version, in which both eyes rotate in the same direction toward an object. The vergence system operates much more slowly than the versional (or turning) system, probably because the synkinetic coordination of vergence with pupillary and accommodative changes acts through smooth intraocular muscles. Disparity vergence is driven by the perception of disparate images of an intended object in the two eyes. The eyes rotate disjunctively so as to superimpose the two images.

The brainstem mechanisms are not as well understood for vergence as for saccades. Stimulation of many areas in the brainstem induces convergence (Bender and Shanzer, 1964), and recordings have been made in the brainstem correlated with convergence motions (Keller and Robinson, 1972), but the exact pathways have not been defined. Since these motions are disjunctive and since the main sequence relationships are different from those of saccades (Stark, 1975; Stark and Bahill, 1979), control of vergence probably involves different pathways from those of saccades.

The usual method of examining vergence evaluates the stationary component, but when vergence must change, it does so by a smooth trajectory. Unlike saccadic motions, the smooth changes of vergence do not suppress visual input or remap space into a stable perceptual space: that is, the world may appear to move during changes of vergence. Of all eye movements, vergence demonstrates the most individual variation. The effects of aging, initial refractive state, or the mechanical tendencies of the eyes to cross or become wall-eyed (esophoria or exophoria) have all been described in the clinical literature.

Some types of VDT use require continual vergence activity as the operator looks back and forth between written and video text at different distances. Also, as the image is refreshed on the VDT, there may be displacement of the letters, which may stimulate disparity vergence. Both kinds of vergence activities might contribute to ocular discomfort.

Changes in the vergence system can often be demonstrated during prolonged performance of a visual task. Luckiesh and Moss (1935a, 1935b) showed that two aspects of the vergence system change with sustained activity. Using reading and inspection tasks lasting up to four hours, they showed that the distance from the observer at which bifixation is no longer possible as the target moves closer is increased with sustained activity. If this near point is expressed in diopters, the parameter is called the amplitude of convergence; consequently, the amplitude of convergence decreases with sustained activity. Luckiesh and Moss also showed that muscle imbalance is increased with prolonged visual activity.

Changes in balance (phorias) were found by Cobb and Moss (1925) to vary in different directions among subjects when one eye was covered and the amount of esophoria or exophoria of the covered nonfixating eye was estimated. The decreased amplitude of convergence caused by visual inspection work was also shown by Brozek and coworkers (1950). Mahto (1972) suggested, on the basis of a small clinical study, that convergence insufficiency is the usual cause of complaints of eyestrain in persons aged 15 to 40 years. The association of close work with these complaints was also noted. The vergence system has been shown to be much more easily disrupted by centrally acting drugs and fatigue than the versional system (Rashbass, 1959; Westheimer and Rashbass, 1961; Westheimer, 1963).[19]

Pupil

Pupil as a Regulator of Light Level The pupil acts as an effective control mechanism for retinal illumination only for small changes of illumination. Larger changes, varying over many log units, are handled by multiple retinal adaptive mechanisms. A more important function of the pupil in regard to VDT studies is that pupil-

---

[19]Double vision is a sensory consequence of alcohol effects on the central nervous system controller of the vergence system.

lary constriction increases depth of focus and hence reduces the need for accommodation. For a presbyopic subject, pupillary constriction may be the major accommodative factor.

A recent study by Cakir and coworkers (1978) has suggested that transient adaptation glare may produce significant transient changes in pupil size in subjects alternately viewing positive- and negative-contrast text projected by a slide projector. They noted that viewing positive-contrast (light characters on a dark background) VDT displays is often alternated with viewing illuminated negative-contrast (dark characters on a light background) hardcopy source documents, and they raised concerns that VDT workers might experience overexposure of their retinas because of alternately looking between the two. Rupp (1981) criticized this study and suggested that the pupillary response may have been caused by the brief period of darkness on the display appearing between the alternating fields. Dainoff (1982) reported that Rupp and coworkers have performed preliminary experiments (using a positive-contrast VDT and an illuminated negative-contrast page of printed material) that confirm Rupp's conjecture. It should also be remembered that transient adaptation does not depend on pupillary changes alone, and changes in threshold have been reported when pupil size is controlled (Boynton, 1961; Rinalducci, 1967). No studies have examined pupillary changes occurring when both VDT display and hard copy have the same (positive or negative) contrast.

Pupillary Constriction Associated with Prolonged Visual Work
Pupillary constriction following prolonged visual work within an institutional setting has been studied by Geacintov and Peavler (1974), who showed a significant pupillary-diameter decrease over the day's work in telephone operators using microfiche or telephone books. This work on pupillary constriction as an indicator of workload should be considered in the context of work on pupillary dilation as an indicator of emotional interest and arousal.

Pupil as a Factor in Visuomotor Discomfort Bartley (1938) showed that slow flicker, 1 to 6 flashes per second, was of too high a frequency to be followed by pupillary movement; instead, a maintained constriction occurred (the Troelstra effect)[20] and

[20]The Troelstra effect (Troelstra, 1968) is a maintained constriction caused by a sequence of light flashes that occur too frequently for the pupillary muscles to follow singly. More recent control studies of the pupil have shown that it can follow at least up to 3 Hz, so that it is not clear whether the static constriction or a small oscillation not indicated by older studies underlies Bartley's results.

discomfort was reported. Halstead (1941) used a mydriatic, scopolamine (which blocks pupillary constriction), when he repeated the Bartley experiment, and under those conditions no ocular strain was reported by the subjects. Fugate and Fry (1956), King (1972), and Fry and King (1975) performed a related experiment. They used very bright light flashes well above sensory threshold and defined a "border between comfort and discomfort"; and because they also believed that pupillary constriction was the source of discomfort, they used atropine to block both the sphincter and ciliary muscles. This approach substantially reduced the reported discomfort in their subjects. These studies implicate an oculomotor mechanism, repetitive pupillary constriction, involved in visual discomfort and further demonstrate relief after eliminating that mechanism by means of drug paralysis. In apparent partial contradiction to these studies, Heaton (1966) found that hyoscine, a mydriatic and blocker of ciliary muscle, did not relieve various complaints of pain with eyestrain. The finding most related to the results of previous investigators was that pain after administration of eserine, a miotic drug, was different but neither greater nor less than that due to eyestrain.

Pupillary Hippus in Relation to Habituation and Sleepiness
Random contractions of the pupil (hippus) are a well-known clinical phenomenon and are present in all normal persons.[21] The amplitude of hippus is largest at moderate pupil sizes and decreases for both large and small values. Large-amplitude hippus has long been associated with a list of vague ailments, and Lowenstein and coworkers (1963) have related this to fatigue in a variety of clinical, normal, and abnormal settings. They point to the possibility of immediate recovery to normal hippus either by instructions to the subject or by psychosensory stimuli.[22] This immediate dishabituation suggests that the fatigue is habituation of central nervous system origin.

Synkinesis of Accommodation, Vergence, and Pupillary Constriction The three mechanisms controlling accommodation, vergence, and pupillary constriction are intimately linked; each is capable of driving the other to some extent. Depth of focus is controlled by

---

[21]Usui and Stark (1978) and others have considered hippus as noise with low band-pass characteristics.
[22]Lowenstein and Loewenfeld (1952) showed a continually diminished responsiveness with fatigue, sleepiness, and boredom. Immediately after a sudden alerting stimulus, they obtained psychosensory dilation of the pupil and increased constriction response to a light flash from subjects.

the pupil moving in synkinesis with accommodation and convergence. In the section on accommodation (see above), it was
pointed out how this asymmetrical interaction between the control
of accommodation and pupillary constriction could reduce the
need for accommodative amplitude.

This triadic synkinesis (O'Neill and Stark, 1968) is an essential
part of the control of accommodation. Vergence drives accommodation (Krishnan et al., 1977), and this has been found to be the
main mechanism for change of focus. Disparity of an intended
stimulus, the binocular parallax that is a signal to the vergence
system, can be detected by the visual system even when the
disparate images are blurred. However, disparity throws the
retinal image off the foveae and thus removes the blur error signal
to accommodation, since blur is only detected via foveal cones.
Thus, in ordinary vision, as in switching attention from a VDT
screen to nearer work or to distance vision, it is not the defocused
images that drive accommodation but the disparate images that
drive vergence. The accommodative state is corrected by
interaction via the vergence-accommodation mechanism.
Accommodation then produces an accommodative pupillary
constriction that increases the depth of focus, which lessens the
requirement for accommodation on a near target. If at this stage
the material on the VDT screen is not sharply focused, the
accommodative system will be stimulated to reduce blur, and the
accommodation-vergence system and the pupillary constriction
system will consequently adjust.

SUMMARY AND CONCLUSIONS

Most of the questions posed at the beginning of this chapter cannot be answered adequately on the basis of existing literature. A
number of studies have reported higher incidences of ocular complaints and temporary alterations in oculomotor functions among
VDT workers than among non-VDT workers. Most of these studies
are flawed, and they do not establish whether these differences
are related to parameters unique to VDT work. These studies have
done little to increase understanding of problems associated with
VDT use and the differences between VDT tasks and other visual
tasks that require prolonged near work.

"Visual fatigue" remains a nebulous concept after many years
of research and discussion (National Research Council, 1939;
Carmichael and Dearborn, 1947). We suggest that it is more
useful to refer to specific phenomena, such as performance
decrement, oculomotor changes, and complaints of visual or ocular
symptoms than loosely to invoke the term "visual fatigue."

Complaints of ocular discomfort or visual symptoms following prolonged near-visual work are by no means unique to VDT workers; some studies suggest, however, that they may be more prevalent among workers who use VDTs than among those who do not. The oculomotor changes reported to follow VDT work are qualitatively similar to those found after other near-visual work; the significance of these changes is not clear. Most of the reviewed studies on oculomotor factors had severe methodological deficits (such as absence of pupillary measurement in testing accommodation), and their results do not support the notion of a specific oculomotor physiological change with prolonged visual work. Even if the numerous suggestive findings are taken at face value as indicating a change in oculomotor state, an important question of interpretation remains. Are these changes a result of "fatigue" or are they a skillful adaptation to the task whereby practice allows effort to be minimized while still permitting adequate performance?

The pupillary constriction experiments are the only studies that point to a specific phenomenon associated with discomfort. Two independent, established investigative groups suggested that drugs that stop pupillary constriction also minimize subjective feelings of discomfort. The relationships between visual task performance, subjective fatigue, oculomotor changes, and motivational and attentional factors remain obscure; careful research that considers all these factors would be required to improve our understanding (see Chapter 10).

8
Job Design and
Organizational Variables

INTRODUCTION

Jobs in which VDTs are used are not purely "VDT jobs," even when
a VDT dominates everything else about the job. A total job is
defined less by the equipment used than by the outcomes to be
achieved, the methods and procedures to be followed, the skills
and abilities demanded, and the general set of circumstances
under which the work is done. Jobs can be carefully designed to
make a work experience satisfying and productive, but they
usually are not; most jobs develop with little real planning, and
any planning that does take place is more likely to consider the
equipment than the person who uses it. If equipment is poorly
designed, constructed, or maintained, a worker is not likely to be
either productive or satisfied; in the extreme example of unsafe
equipment, a worker's complaints are likely to anticipate health
and safety hazards. Even equipment that is poor but not physically dangerous can negatively affect mental health or the sense
of well-being and, perhaps, job performance.

Workers' Complaints and Job Structures

VDTs, like any other work technology, can be used properly or
improperly. The research evidence examined in previous chapters
has indicated little likelihood that VDT use involves serious health
or safety hazards, but there is evidence that some jobs in which
VDTs are central parts of the work equipment are associated with
many kinds of worker complaints--including (but not only) complaints related to vision. On some jobs, including some where
visual contact with a display unit is relatively intensive, complaints seem rare. Although it may be that the number of complaints is related to the quality of VDT equipment, there has not
been any research testing that hypothesis. In the absence of such

research showing a substantial difference across equipment in performance decrements on a standard task, for example, it seems more useful to consider whether the design of a job as a whole is associated with the variations in complaints. Perhaps some aspects of jobs are associated with VDT technology but are not necessary concomitants of VDT use: an example would be the availability of immediate feedback (from either the work or the supervisor or both) about productivity. Perhaps other aspects of the job, such as low status, close supervision, or absence of opportunity to plan work sequences, lead to dissatisfaction and health problems independently of whether there is a VDT involved in a job.

We note that complaints are less likely to be reported by workers in "good" jobs--those in which a worker is well paid, has had substantial training or education, and has varied kinds and levels of responsibility (National Institute for Occupational Safety and Health, 1981; Smith et al., 1981). Rather, most of the complaints are reported by workers in jobs in which a single task (e.g., data entry) dominates the workday, the pay is relatively low, and a worker's responsibility is almost entirely limited to working continually and avoiding errors. Such jobs are not ordinarily described as good; indeed they can be seen as deadly jobs in the sense that they seem to stifle, if not kill, human initiative, creativity, and sense of achievement. The question that demands answering is whether people who complain and develop various symptoms--including visual or musculoskeletal discomfort, physiological changes, or dissatisfaction with the job--are responding to the equipment, the basic nature of the job, or their own perception of the job and its opportunities and limitations.

Complaints exist. They must be taken seriously by researchers. Should the response simply be concentrated efforts to find causal relationships between characteristics of VDT equipment and visual complaints or problems? We think not: it seems unlikely that such an approach, by itself, will offer the greatest probability of payoff in terms of human well-being. Rather, we believe that research should also consider total job design.

No systematic research program has yet been undertaken to study job design specifically for jobs in which VDTs are used. Consequently, there is no adequate body of knowledge concerning the psychosocial aspects of VDT work and the resulting mental and physical strains (see Table 2.1 in Chapter 2 for an evaluation of existing studies). Studies have not examined the wide array of psychosocial stressors that can influence how VDTs are used and how their use may influence workers' well-being. However, there has been research that shows the kinds of psychosocial stressors that affect employee well-being in other kinds of situations.

Work on psychosocial stressors in jobs, and particularly work
that emphasizes the desirability of a good fit of the characteristics of the job and the characteristics of the worker, seems very
much worth considering in evaluating complaints about VDTs.
Accordingly, this chapter identifies the kinds of psychosocial
characteristics of jobs that have been associated with employee
well-being in other kinds of work, offers what might be called a
pretheoretical point of view about some of the relationships
among these characteristics, and indicates how such characteris-
istics can be considered in designing jobs and research in order to
eliminate or reduce workers' complaints and symptoms of physical
and mental problems.

Defining Psychosocial Stress and Strain

Strains refer to complaints and include negative affective states
or changes in attitude, performance decrements, and poor biological functioning. Strains often result from stressors, including
stressors on the job. Most of the literature on the psychogenic
aspects of work that effect strains focuses on emotional states
and physiological responses (e.g., heart rate, cholesterol level, and
blood pressure). Strains are usually not diseases themselves, but
may be risk factors for mental or physical illnesses. In many
cases, a link between a condition of the work environment and
those risk factors may have health consequences that are poorly
understood. For example, is one's life really shortened if one has
a heated argument with a coworker that raises one's blood
pressure for a few minutes? Is an elevated heart rate due to anger
unhealthy but an elevated heart rate due to working on a complex
arithmetic problem not (or less) unhealthy? As for the health
consequences of emotional reactions to work, although one does
not expect work life to be euphoric, workers probably prefer to
experience satisfaction rather than dissatisfaction with their job
and a sense of psychological well-being rather than feelings of
anxiety, depression, and anger. The reader should keep this
discussion in mind when evaluating the review of literature that
follows.

Objective job stress (or stressors) refers to conditions of the
work environment that represent some demand (such as, workload)
on a person's abilities or represent some deficit of supplies or
resources (such as salary, praise, opportunities to participate) to
meet some need of the employee. Subjective job stressors refers
to an employee's perceptions and reports of these environmental
conditions.

This chapter focuses on psychosocial rather than physical
stressors. Physical stressors refers to the direct physical effects

of physical forces (mechanical, heat, light, and chemical, for example) on psychological and physiological well-being; psycho-social stressors refers to the symbolic meaning of actions and of conditions of the environment. Psychosocial stressors may come from several sources, including the design of the job (such as pacing, control over tasks, sequencing, quantity, and nature of tasks), the psychosocial environment of work (such as the degree of supportive relations with superiors, peers, and subordinates), and the broader organizational system (such as the reward and influence structures and the isolation of the person from fiscal and political turbulence in the larger environment of which the organization is a part).

A FRAMEWORK FOR STUDYING PSYCHOSOCIAL STRESSORS IN VDT WORK

Person-Environment Fit

We find it useful to think of the misfit between the characteristics of a worker and of the work environment as a potential precursor of psychological and physiological strain. This concept of misfit is used here as a heuristic device for evaluating the extent to which VDT technology, the social environments in which VDTs are used, and the nature of the human operator contribute to health-related outcomes. The basic hypothesis is that the goodness of fit between characteristics of a person (P) and the environment (E) can be thought of as a predictor of well-being (see, e.g., French and Kahn, 1962; Levi, 1972; French et al., 1974) and performance (McGrath, 1976). By considering both a VDT operator and the work environment, one can start to explain situations in which one worker is overwhelmed by a task that does not overwhelm another person, as well as situations that are likely to overwhelm or not to overwhelm most workers. It is noteworthy that with one exception (Johansson and Aronsson, 1980), none of the studies of psychosocial stressors in VDT work (summarized in Table 2.1) even mentions the possible contribution of personal characteristics to health outcomes.

We can think about two kinds of goodness of P-E fit in work situations (French, et al., 1974). The first is the fit between the person's needs (or preferences, desires, values, etc.) and the related supplies for these needs in the job environment. A variety of needs might be thought about in terms of person-environment fit, such as needs for cognitive stimulation, for social support or social interaction, for structure and clarity in task definition and task demands, for esteem, and for achievement. Many of these needs are discussed in more detail below with regard to VDT work.

A second type of fit is concerned with the match between demands in the job environment and the relevant person's abilities to meet those demands. For example, one can think of the fit between the demands of a VDT job for accuracy and speed and a person's ability to do such work with accuracy and speed.

These two kinds of fit, needs-supplies and demands-abilities, may not always represent two mutually exclusive classifications. Excessive job demands, for example, may threaten a worker who has strong security needs as much as one who has inadequate abilities. Nevertheless, the distinction is used as a reminder that dimensions of fit must be considered both from the viewpoint of an employee's characteristics and motives and from the viewpoint of a job's demands.

Objective and Subjective Fit

The concept of P-E fit also distinguishes between objective and subjective fit. Objective P and objective E are operationally defined as P and E measured free of any bias in self-reporting. Subjective P and E refer to the perceptions of these parameters by the person (employee); consequently, they are measurable only by self-reporting. Subjective fit is expected to be related to objective fit, but the relationship can be less than perfect. The relationship can be weakened by a person's subjective distortions (e.g., defense mechanisms such as denial and repression) or by lack of information about the objective state of P or E because such information may be hard to provide or intentionally withheld.

Although objective misfit may have to be changed in order to improve the objective conditions of work, the pathway by which the reduction of such misfit reduces psychogenic ill-being is hypothesized to be partly and significantly through a worker's perceptions of the misfit. This hypothesis is supported by the work of Kraut (1965), French and Caplan (1972), and Frankenhaeuser (1980) and is an important point in both theory and application. If a well-intended change in work conditions is not perceived as such, an objective improvement in work conditions will unintentionally generate strain. For example, the introduction of VDTs to make a work environment quieter and to make text editing more pleasant may be negatively perceived by employees because it generates a misfit with regard to their technological word-processing skills. Rather than feeling more satisfied, the employees may feel just the opposite, at least until their objective skills change. To take another example, a VDT operator may perceive good fit with the job ("I key in 300 characters per minute; the job only requires that I key in 250"), when the objective fit is poor (the real typing speed of the person is only 250; and the job actually requires a speed of 400, but this has not been pointed out to the VDT operator). In terms of person-environment fit, the two characteristics of a person, needs and abilities, along with the two characteristics of the environment, supplies and demands, combine to determine how the ways in which VDTs are used in the workplace affect workers' well-being.[1]

STRESSORS FOR STUDY IN VDT WORK

Given the paucity and inconclusiveness of the psychosocial literature on VDTs, one can only suggest possible stressors for study. The stressors discussed below were selected primarily because of circumstantial evidence or because other research on psychosocial stressors has suggested that they may have important and general effects on workers' well-being.

Control

The amount of control a worker has may have an important influence on stress in VDT-related work. Control can be exercised over the onset of a specific stressor, its intensity, its termination, or any combination of these (Cohen, 1980). In studying VDT use, researchers might examine the extent to which an operator can control (a) the introduction into the workplace of the specific hardware or software itself and the alteration of his or her role in using the new technology; (b) the amount of incoming work and associated deadlines; (c) the variety of the work content (such as data entry, data acquisition, or some mix; complex as well as simple interactive tasks; etc.); (d) the amount of time spent continuously at the VDT and the scheduling of such time (such as massed versus spaced periods of time), and interactions with other persons (such as telephone and in-person interruptions). It should be clear from this list, which is not exhaustive, that "control" is not a unitary concept; there are many aspects of VDT work to be examined from the perspective of control.

---

[1] It is not our intent to advocate the concept of P-E fit as the particular device for studying VDTs and well-being; rather, it is meant as an example and is meant to provide a framework for discussing job design. Readers interested in empirical research involving the theory may consult a number of references (e.g., Harrison, 1976; Kulka, 1979; Caplan, 1983).

Opportunity to Control: E

In the studies on VDT use reported in Table 2.1 in Chapter 2, some employees have complained about lack of control and others have not. Rigid pacing of a job task by a VDT and automatic monitoring of the rate and accuracy of task performance are among the concerns expressed by VDT workers about control (Johansson and Aronsson, 1980). Equipment-paced work, in general, has usually been found to be more likely to produce undesirable emotional and somatic symptoms when compared with self-paced work (Caplan et al., 1975; French et al., 1982). The research to date does not permit firm conclusions about how variations in control influence employee well-being when work involves VDT use, but research on control per se suggests that there are measurable, undesirable effects on employee well-being. Literature reviewed by Cohen (1980) suggests that lack of control may produce emotional and physiological strain as well as performance deficits and insensitivity to the needs of others. Many of these outcomes may, in turn, adversely affect the well-being of other employees, starting a chain reaction of strains and other stressors. For example, highly controlled jobs, such as machine-paced assembly work, can produce elevated adrenalin and noradrenalin levels (Frankenhaeuser and Gardell, 1976). Such jobs may also lead to anxiety, depression, boredom, and somatic complaints (Caplan et al., 1980; French et al., 1982).

Need for Control: P

Individual differences in need for control are important. Experiments by Lundberg and Frankenhaeuser (1978) suggest that withdrawal of control, or low levels of control, are particularly upsetting for people with a high need for control (Burger and Cooper, 1979). Among those with high needs for control are Type A coronary-prone people. Experiments show that in uncontrollable situations, Type A people have particularly high autonomic reactivity (Glass, 1977). It is hypothesized that this reactivity may increase the risk of atherosclerosis. If so, VDT work that threatens a person's need for control could increase the risk of coronary heart disease. Reactivity to uncontrollable aspects of VDT work may vary by gender as well as by personality type. In a sample of Swedish workers, Frankenhaeuser (1980) found that females had lower catecholamine reactivity than males to uncontrollable stressors, suggesting that females are better able to withstand exposure to jobs involving such tasks.

These data suggest that lack of control may produce strain and that there may be individual differences in strain responsivity depending on the person's need for control. (The extent to which too much control can be a stressor is discussed below.) As noted, there are a variety of points at which control can be exercised in VDT work. Distinguishing among those points when assessing the role of control in VDT work may allow specific enough diagnoses of the stressors so that preventive or corrective action can be designed.

Participation

Participation, a concept closely related to control, refers to having a say in decisions that affect the nature of one's work. In VDT work, participation could extend to decisions regarding the introduction of VDT work into the job, the flow and nature of the work to be processed, and the nature of the VDT hardware and software.

Opportunity to Participate: E

Cross-cultural surveys in the United States, Italy, Yugoslavia, and Israel indicate that greater perceived control is associated with greater job satisfaction (Tannenbaum et al., 1974). Multivariate cross-sectional analyses suggest that participation may reduce job dissatisfaction and boredom, allowing employees to influence person-environment fit on a number of facets of work, including task complexity, responsibility, and quantitative workload (Caplan et al., 1980; French et al., 1982). Consequently, participation may be a useful social mechanism for reducing such strain in VDT work when misfit is present in the job.

Need to Participate: P

People's need to participate has not been well studied; see the discussion above regarding need for control.

Predictability and Controllability

Unpredictable events are by definition uncontrollable in terms of when their onset will occur, but not all uncontrollable events are unpredictable. For example, a VDT user may know in advance that a computer system serving the VDT will be down for a specified period and that the user will be unable to do anything about it. One of the special aspects of VDT work is unpredictable system breakdown. In time-sharing systems, delays in access, processing, and output may be both unpredictable and uncontrollable in that one cannot influence when these delays will occur.

Unpredictable Events: E

Overall, little research has been done on the effects of unpredictable versus predictable stressors. Johansson and Aronsson (1980) had data on six VDT operators who, fortunately (for the study), encountered an unexpected system breakdown and showed elevated levels of adrenalin, systolic and diastolic blood pressure, heart rate, irritation, feelings of fatigue, and boredom. Laboratory research examining the role of unpredictable noise as a stressor found that it had no effect on performance (Glass and Singer, 1972; Gardner, 1978). Unfortunately, these studies confound unpredictability and uncontrollability. However, studies of warnings before disasters suggest that people cope better when they have warning even though they cannot control the onset and effects of the disaster (see, e.g., Janis and Mann, 1977).

Tolerance of Unpredictability: P

Experiments giving people realistic job previews indicate that such previews reduce job turnover as well as increase job satisfaction (see, e.g., Ilgen and Seeley, 1974; Wanous, 1978). Whether such previews have their effects because they make the job predictable or because of other mechanisms (such as creating feelings of trust or opportunities for better selection in and out of the job by prospective job applicants) is not known. Research could be done to determine the extent to which strains might be reduced by giving VDT operators and those who make demands on them realistic expectations about system reliability. By increasing people's expectations of unpredictability, one might increase their tolerance of it. No research on this topic in VDT work has been done.

As with control, predictability can be influenced at several points in the flow of VDT work. Some strategies for experimentally reducing strain might focus on changing P (such as increasing tolerance for unpredictability); other strategies might just as easily focus on making the design of the work environment better fit a person. For example, the flow of work to a VDT operator could be made more predictable by improving the reliability of VDT systems, carefully training those who provide work for the VDT operator, and studying workflow patterns. Even an impending peak in workload might be better tolerated if a VDT operator were given plenty of early warning to allow adjustments to be made in other pending work. Experiments that vary such parameters, as well as studies that assess the predictability of different aspects of VDT-related work rather than characterize job predictability at a global level, are needed. Such studies may lead to knowledge about how to estimate the strain-producing contributions of different parts of the workflow and how to locate points, if any, of intervention.

Complexity

The complexity of work performed using a VDT can vary dramatically, from that of a programmer or scientist attempting to create or discover new algorithms to that of a clerical worker confined to entering meaningless (to the operator) data (such as strings of invoice numbers run together on a code sheet).

Studying complexity in VDT-related work is likely to be complicated. It would be ideal to define and measure complexity in terms of standard units of cognitive information load. This ideal can be met in the laboratory (Berlyne, 1958), where an investigator can carefully define "bits of information" and can carefully vary the presentation (e.g., complexity of a visual pattern) of stimuli to a viewer. In the workplace, however, the problem of comparing different types of work in terms of bits of information remains unsolved. As an example, how should a secretary doing word processing have workload defined in terms of bits of information? What constitutes a bit in information theory when comparing the work of entering first-draft text and of making revisions? If the secretary's phone rings while VDT work is being done, is the interruption included as part of the normal definition of complexity as bits of information? And so on.

Recognizing this problem, social scientists have tended to define complexity in the work environment in terms of a number of stressors: (a) relatively vague definitions of the occupational role (role ambiguity); (b) changes in tasks from day to day (variety); (c) contact with people (which may involve unpredictability, uncontrollability, and variety); (d) time sharing rather than linear processing of multiple role responsibilities; and (e) work with several groups outside one's own immediate work group (Kohn and Schooler, 1969; Caplan et al., 1980). A VDT job might be defined as complex with only a few of these elements present in almost any combination. For example, a mathematician at a VDT might have little contact with people (simplicity), a relatively vague definition of the job and of work from day to day (complexity), and task variety across time—some days routine and some days involving a high level of problem solving (complexity).

These elements of complexity have not been examined in any systematic way as components of jobs involving VDTs. Some of the studies discussed in Table 2.1 in Chapter 2 compare VDT operators whose occupations look as though they might vary in level of complexity, requirements for cognitive skills and knowledge, and the level of complexity desired by employees. In such studies the extent to which employee (person) versus task (environment) characteristics account for group differences in well-being cannot be determined because no differentiation between these characteristics has been made. The separate elements of complexity also have not been examined in VDT studies, so the effect of complexity in VDT work on well- being is unknown.

Although research on complexity and well-being has not been conducted on VDT-related work, it has been done in a wide variety of occupations. The studies indicate that complexity can affect employee well-being. In a cross-sectional survey study of over 2,000 employees in 23 different occupations ranging from unskilled work to highly skilled professions (Harrison, 1976; Caplan et al., 1980), poor P-E fit on job complexity was associated with emotional strain and somatic complaints (such as heart beating hard, sweaty palms, and trouble sleeping). It is important to note that too little as well as too much complexity produced these outcomes. When one considered only the absolute level of complexity in the job (E) or only the absolute level of desired complexity (P), the findings were not as striking.

Lack of complexity--i.e., repetitive, monotonous work--has been found to be a key predictor of job dissatisfaction in a number of studies in the United States, some of which were of random samples of the U.S. workforce, and in Scandinavia (see, e.g., Walker and Guest, 1952; Gardell, 1971; Barnowe et al., 1973). With regard to physical health, research in Scandinavia suggests that lack of complexity in work can increase the risk of accidents, headaches and nervous disturbances, and abnormal catecholamine excretion, although the results of this study are themselves complex (Johansson et al., 1978).[2]

Too much complexity, as aptly characterized by the Peter Principle (Peter and Hull, 1969), is believed to lead to feelings of incompetence, emotional strain, and poor performance. Aside from the study of 23 occupations, discussed above (Harrison, 1976; Caplan et al., 1980), very little is known about excess complexity in tasks. But it is a very important concept when studying

---

[2]The interested reader is advised to consider the findings in their entirety. They deal with how different aspects of complex and noncomplex tasks may affect different physiological and emotional responses, a case of response specificity.

changes in work technology. The move per se from non-VDT to VDT technology may appear to future VDT operators as a significant increase in complexity even if, from the point of view of those who designed the hardware and software, the VDT will "greatly simplify things." Once an employee becomes familiar with the new technology, however, the perception of excess complexity may disappear.

Anecdotal evidence (e.g., Leo, 1980) indicates that fear of computers and allied technology may occur because the machines are viewed as "too complicated." These fears seem to know no boundaries of occupation and can be found in executive as well as in line positions. We do not know how widespread such fear is and what effect it has on physical and mental health when VDTs are introduced. It would seem useful to conduct systematic research on the magnitude of such effects and the educational conditions that might overcome such fears. It is likely that these effects are secular. Younger people, increasingly exposed to VDT technology in school and recreation, will probably have fewer problems accepting VDT technology in work than will older people.

The rate at which elements of a job become more complex has been referred to as complexification. Large-scale, ecological analyses suggest that as complexification increases in societies, so does mental illness, suicide, and bankruptcy (Terreberry, 1968). Toffler (1970) argues that "future shock" consists of a high rate of complexification without the resources to adapt to it. If this is the case in VDT work, then it would be valuable to monitor the rate of change in VDT software and hardware technology as a predictor of the well-being of employees. To our knowledge no such research has been done.

Role Ambiguity

Role ambiguity refers to the extent to which a given work role is clearly defined for an employee. Cross-sectional correlational analyses indicate that too much ambiguity relative to a person's preferred level of clarity-ambiguity is associated with job dissatisfaction, depression, anxiety, and anger-irritation (Harrison, 1978).

Role ambiguity may be pervasive in the workforce (Kahn et al., 1964), but of 33 facets of work, role ambiguity ranked in the lower one-third in its effects on job satisfaction in multivariate analyses of data from a random sample of the U.S. workforce (Barnowe et al., 1973). Lack of challenge and lack of complexity were the most important causes of occupational strain. Is role ambiguity an important stressor in VDT-related work? The variable has not been studied in VDT-related work. Any effects of too little ambiguity in highly structured, input-oriented clerical VDT work may be highly correlated with lack of task complexity and variety. There is no evidence of any association between role ambiguity, per se, and physical health outcomes (see Caplan et al., 1980).

Threat of Unemployment

Some VDT research (e.g., Johansson and Aronsson, 1980) has found that VDT operators, particularly those in clerical occupations, worry about the possibility that their jobs might be eliminated in the future by a computer. How might such worry affect the well-being of these operators?

We know of one study of the effect of the threat of job loss and the actual job loss on physical and mental well-being (Cobb and Kasl, 1977); it followed employees from the time of the announced job loss to two years after termination. As evidenced by higher levels of anxiety and serum cholesterol, the anticipation period was more stressful than the time of actual termination. Lazarus (1966) reviews other literature suggesting that the threat of an unpleasant event is more strain-producing than the actual event. No research has assessed the prevalence and strength of threatened job loss perceived in various VDT jobs in relationship to physiological and psychological manifestations of strain. Consequently, we cannot draw conclusions about its effects on well-being in VDT work.

Quantitative Workload

Up to this point we have considered qualitative aspects of the work. Is it controllable? How complex is it? And so on. There is also the factor of quantitative workload, the sheer amount of work to be done in a given unit of time regardless of its qualitative nature. The pace and flow of work are important aspects of quantitative workload.

A study in Sweden (Johansson and Aronsson, 1980) presents evidence suggesting that the nature of the human use of VDT technology influences the level of workload over the course of the day. This study showed that the heaviest use of computer systems occurs in the afternoon and that with increased use there are greater delays in response time by the VDT in interactive and batch modes and greater probabilities of unscheduled breakdowns in the system. Johansson and Aronsson note that VDT workers appear to cope with this pattern by increasing the pace at which they work in the morning: the increased pace in the morning is insurance against system delays in the afternoon. This self-pacing appears to lead to elevated adrenalin levels in the morning. The data are not precise enough to indicate the extent to which the elevation of adrenalin precedes the anticipation of high workload or results from the high workload itself. Furthermore, the health consequences of these elevations are unknown.

In a longitudinal study of a 21-day planned (i.e., anticipated, predictable) computer shutdown at a large university, there was evidence that the workload generated in anticipation of the shutdown was more likely to lead to anxiety and to elevated heart rates among people who had traits like those of the Type A coronary-prone person (Caplan and Jones, 1975). These people have an inner sense of time urgency, a tendency to express preferences for competitive situations, and a preference for deadline pressures. Later work by Glass (1977) suggested that the elevated levels of anxiety and heart rate may have been part of a reaction to threatened, strong needs for control that characterize Type A persons. Such research suggests that there may be individual differences in response to workload pressures created by VDTs. It may be important to assess the extent to which excessive quantitative workload (E) signals a threat to some operators' strong needs for control but poses no threat to others for whom this need is not as salient (P).

Laboratory research indicates that quantitative overload (E > P) can increase serum cholesterol levels and maintain high pulse rates (Sales, 1969) and that both too little (E < P) and too much work (E > P) can increase noradrenalin and adrenalin (Frankenhaeuser et al., 1971; Frankenhaeuser and Gardell, 1976). Field studies have found similar effects of deadline pressures on the cholesterol levels of medical students facing academic exams (e.g., Horwitz and Bronte-Stewart, 1962), on tax accountants approaching the April federal income tax deadline (Friedman et al., 1958), and among professional staff at the National Aeronautics and Space Administration, whose telephone calls and meetings were observed and tallied (French and Caplan, 1972). There is also evidence that heavy quantitative workload may disrupt the circadian rhythm of adrenal cortisol (Caplan et al., 1979). Such effects may occur in VDT-related work that involves poor P-E fit on workload.

Multivariate analyses of stressors in data from a national sample survey of the workforce (Barnowe et al., 1973) indicate that workload, per se, ranks near the bottom of 33 facets predictive of job dissatisfaction. The analyses suggest that it is not hard work itself that is the key stressor on effects; rather, the culprit may be excessive workload that is also uncontrollable or carries with it misfit with regard to complexity. This analysis is confirmed by results of a study of 23 occupations that showed the effects on psychological strain (such as depression and anxiety) of

P-E misfit on quantitative workload were greater for persons who also had P-E misfit on job complexity, either too little or too much complexity (Caplan et al., 1980; French et al., 1982). Persons with the right amount of complexity in their work relative to what they wanted were the least affected by large amounts of work, even when the workload exceeded their preferred levels. Overall, these findings suggest that the study of VDT operations should consider both the quantitative and qualitative nature of the workload.

Prescription for Overload—Deadline Plus Delay

We have discussed both delays and deadlines as potential stressors in VDT work. Together they can greatly increase quantitative overload. Deadlines create quantitative workloads by setting a time limit during which a given amount of work must be accomplished; delays exacerbate the pressure of a deadline, reducing the amount of time for completing the job.

There is some evidence of individual differences in tolerance for delays (P). Type A persons tend to be impatient (Friedman and Rosenman, 1959). Furthermore, Type A coronary-prone persons are described as having a sense of time urgency—a sense that no matter how much time there is, it is never quite enough. In studies of VDT workers, Johansson and Aronsson (1980) found that operators preferred having delays of less than 5 seconds when awaiting a system reply to a VDT input. If Type A persons are faced with delays they feel are excessive, they might be more upset than Type B persons by the delay. Research by Glass (1977) indicates that Type A people have a strong need for control. Long delays on a VDT are periods during which an operator gives up control to the machine; for Type A people, the longer the delay, the more the need for control may be threatened. It may be the loss of control, rather than the quantitative workload, that is especially strain-producing about VDT delays, but stress research on the health consequences of these delays, short of a computer breakdown, has not been reported.

In general, the meaning of poor P-E fit on workload to the VDT operator may be important to assess before attempting to determine the effects of such misfit on strain. Delays induced by computer system overloading may not be as threatening to a scientist faced with only vague and perhaps self-imposed deadlines as they are to a newspaper reporter attempting to meet a press deadline. And overload in VDT-related work may signal to some VDT users that their work is important and, consequently, that their VDT-related jobs are secure; in contrast, underload may signal a possible reduction in workforce.

Responsibility for Persons

Some jobs involving VDTs--for example, air traffic control work--
also involve direct responsibility for the lives and well-being of
other people. Given that fact, is it possible that the responsibility
and not the VDT exposure produces strain? Might the two factors
have joint effects? Although no studies of VDT work have considered responsibility as a competing stressor, there is enough
literature linking responsibility to ill-being to justify serious
consideration.

Responsibility: E

Research suggests that responsibility for persons plays a role in
the development of coronary heart disease (see, e.g., Russek,
1965). Studies of foremen and people in jobs involving both
responsibility for persons and role conflicts, have shown that they
are particularly prone to peptic ulcer (see, e.g., Doll and Jones,
1951; Gosling, 1958; Pflanz et al., 1966). Of particular interest is
the study by Cobb and Rose (1973) of the universe of U. S.
medical records of air traffic controllers and commercial pilots,
all of whom entered their occupations passing the similar
standardized medical examinations. The data (corrected for age
effects) showed that of the two occupational groups, air traffic
controllers had developed the highest incidence of high blood
pressure and peptic ulcer. Furthermore, the disease rates were
highest for controllers at airports with high-density, compared
with low-density, air traffic. The data do not allow one to isolate
the extent to which these occupational differences in illness
represent effects caused by quantitative workload, complexity, or
responsibility for persons.

Responsibility: P

With regard to coronary heart disease, Kasl (1978) notes that some
large sample epidemiological surveys have shown that employees
at higher levels of management have lower levels of coronary
heart disease (e.g., Lee and Schneider, 1958; Pell and d'Alonzo,
1963). This finding runs contrary to the responsibility hypothesis.
Perhaps responsibility (E) is not the key stressor, but rather
whether the amount of responsibility exceeds one's resources (P).
Individual differences in preference for responsibility and in need
to discharge responsibility (P) versus supplies of authority and
resources to meet that need (E) have rarely been examined. One
study found that too little as well as too much responsibility (P-E

misfit) was associated with high levels of cholesterol. Neither the amount of responsibility desired (P) nor the amount demanded (E) predicted high levels of cholesterol (Caplan, 1971; French et al., 1974). This finding has not been replicated.

Given the possibility that responsibility for persons may affect employee well-being, this aspect of work should probably be measured in studies of VDT operations in which such responsibility varies as part of the task. In this way, one could statistically control for psychosocial effects of responsibility when exploring any link between exposure to the physical aspects of VDTs and health.

Role Conflict

Conflicting demands from different persons in one's work does not seem like an obvious concomitant of VDT work. Should it be suspected in some VDT operations, there is literature on it from other work situations (e.g., Kahn et al., 1964; Kahn and Quinn, 1970; Miles, 1976). Its main effects appear to be job-related tension (Kahn et al., 1964) and anger-irritation (Caplan et al., 1980).

Social Support

Social support can be defined as affirmation of someone's attitudes and beliefs, liking, trust and respect, and certain kinds of direct assistance (Katz and Kahn, 1978). There are a variety of other definitions (see Caplan, 1979), but they generally share the above properties. Some VDT work may, by its organization, reduce social interaction and thereby reduce opportunities for social support among workers. We have already noted that, at least in theory, certain types of stressors can occur as part of the way in which VDT-related work is organized (heavy or excessive workload, boring work that lacks adequate complexity, and so on). If the design of a job reduces chances for social support, the undesirable effects of VDT work on well-being may be magnified.

Evidence suggests that loss of social support reduces well-being both directly and via its effect as a buffer between stressors and workers. Having a nonsupportive supervisor in the workplace has been associated with increased risk of mortality from coronary heart disease (Medalie, et al., 1973). Lack of social support at work has also been associated with dissatisfaction with work and with depression (see, e.g., Caplan et al., 1980).

When stressors such as those that have been described above are present in the work environment (heavy workload, excessive

responsibility, too little control, etc.), social support may buffer
their effects on well-being. Buffering refers to interaction:
social support reduces the relationship between the stressor and
health consequence. Buffering has been found with regard to a
number of health-related outcomes (see reviews by Cobb, 1976;
House, 1981). These outcomes include serum cholesterol
elevations among employees losing their jobs (Cobb and Kasl,
1977; Gore, 1978), escapist drinking among a national random
sample of employees experiencing various levels of occupational
stressors,[3] emotional strain in a sample of 23 occupations ranging
from blue to white collar (LaRocco et al., 1980), and ulcer
symptoms among factory workers (House and Wells, 1978). In
other studies (such as Pinneau, 1975; Frydman, 1981), however,
social support has not buffered the effects of stressors on strain.

Although the conditions under which buffering does and does
not occur are not understood, the evidence of both the direct and
buffering effects of social support on well-being suggests that it is
an important health-related predictor. In VDT-related work,
social support takes the form of supervision as well as relationships with peers and with any clients who interact with the VDT
user. Accordingly, studies of VDT-related work may encounter
health-related outcomes that are partly affected by the social
support available to the VDT user. By studying that support, it
would be possible to determine the extent to which VDT work
generates certain types of interpersonal frictions and generates
needs for social support as a buffer. It would be possible to
determine the extent to which any lack of social support is not
unique to the VDT work, but is part of the larger organizational
climate of the worksite.

When studying the role of social support in VDT-related work
as a buffer of strain or, when low, as a stressor, it may be useful
to view supervisory support in terms of two major factors that
have been repeatedly identified in leadership studies. These
factors can be generally described as task and process orientation
(see, e.g., Bales, 1950; Bowers and Seashore, 1966; House and
Mitchell, 1975). Task orientation, sometimes called initiating
structure, deals with supervision that provides information to a
subordinate about the definition and execution of the work role.
Process orientation, sometimes called consideration, refers to the
provision to the subordinate of mutual trust, respect, consideration for feelings, and general rapport (Stodgill, 1974). A review of
the literature (House and Mitchell, 1975) indicates that employees

---

[3]Robert P. Quinn, associate research scientist, Institute for Social
Research, University of Michigan, personal communication, 1973.

in some jobs want task leadership more than process leadership, while in other jobs the reverse may be true, and in still other jobs some more equal mix may be desired. Following House's theory (House and Mitchell, 1975), in particularly noncomplex work, such as that involving highly repetitive VDT input of data, employees may experience more satisfaction with the job if the supervisor is process oriented, because there is little in the way of task information and structure that is required (or perhaps that can be changed). The best a supervisor can do under such circumstances is to provide a pleasant and agreeable environment as compensation for the potential stress of an uninteresting job. In highly professional VDT-related work, such as the work of scientists and engineers, however, VDT operators may want task orientation-- that is, technical information. In such jobs, satisfaction derives primarily from structural and informational guidance and from the intrinsic nature of the job, not from leadership that is aimed at creating a pleasant social environment. Thus, the extent to which a style of supervision leads to VDT operator satisfaction may depend on whether that style meets the needs of the operator, which probably vary by type of VDT work. Person-environment fit with regard to social support, rather than either amount of support (E) or amount desired (P) may be an important predictor of strain.

Is there anything about the physical parameters of VDT work that might influence social support? In highly computerized environments, it is possible (although it need not be) for VDT employees to be denied the social support that can derive from interaction with coworkers and others. For example, in the interest of reducing glare, cubicles may be erected that block off vision in all directions except to the screen. In highly computerized operations, even some forms of supervisory feedback, particularly negative feedback, may come to the employee in the form of computer-generated messages, sometimes called error messages (such communication, even if containing words of praise, does not constitute true social support because it lacks the element of human response). Such situations and the extent to which a task is highly confined to a terminal itself when deadlines and other pressures arise may reduce opportunities for social support and may deny people the opportunity to satisfy basic needs for social interaction (Murray, 1938).

There has been no systematic study of the extent to which different types of VDT work have an effect on social support. Given the key role of social support in the literature on psychosocial stressors and well-being, it may be worthwhile to investigate whether VDT work in some conditions creates a new form of sociotechnical system (Emery and Trist, 1960) with important effects on employee well-being.

DISCUSSION AND CONCLUSIONS

The VDT, like the typewriter, is a technology that can be used in ways that abuse or augment the human resources of society. In this chapter we have attempted to indicate the types of stressors that might be associated with VDT work when the work is not organized with the well-being of the user in mind.

In our opinion, most, if not all, of the stressors we have reviewed (unlike the physical properties of the VDT itself) are not inherent to VDT technology and software but depend on how the VDT work is structured. Therefore, there is a great deal of freedom to make work at a VDT as pleasurable or as painful as work at a desk with a typewriter. If there are health risks inherent in VDT work that derive from psychosocial stressors, there is no compelling evidence in the literature. As reviewed earlier, the VDT literature on psychosocial stressors is, with a few exceptions, inconclusive because the designs of the studies have not allowed conclusiveness.

VDT use occurs in jobs that vary greatly in their complexity, responsibility for others, quantitative workload, control over the work pace, and so on. Consequently, it would be accurate to conclude that there is no such thing as VDT work if it is defined as a particular occupational title or condition. The concept of VDT work is relatively meaningless for use in studies of occupational health because the concept refers to too diverse a set of conditions. Systematic studies of the relative contributions of each psychosocial stressor as a component of the context in which the VDT is used would provide a much greater increase in knowledge about the psychogenic health effects of VDT use than would studies that compare a VDT group and a non-VDT group, as has been done in some designs.

If more detailed evaluations of psychogenic factors in VDT work and well-being are carried out, P-E fit theory may provide a useful conceptual device for systematically examining the relationship of the VDT user and the work environment to user well-being. The concept of P-E fit can help generate the options for improving fit between a person and a job and can involve both changes in the person (selection, training, and so on) and in the environment (managerial and coworker increase in resources, workflow, variety, complexity, increased opportunity for participation, and so on). Once areas of misfit are identified, one can turn to choices between how much of P and how much of E should be changed. Some of the strategies for reducing stressors have been discussed elsewhere (e.g., French and Caplan, 1972; Caplan et al., 1980; French et al., 1982) as well as the strategies for introducing change (e.g., Bowers and Hauser, 1977; Katz and Kahn, 1978). The selection of P or E (or a mix) as the target for improving P-E fit in VDT work in which misfit exists should necessarily consider both the acceptance of the strategy by the VDT user as well as the costs of the strategy in terms of human well-being. Acceptance is relatively easy to assess; assessing costs may be quite another matter. But it is that assessment that is at the heart of research on psychosocial stressors and how they affect employee well-being. It is that assessment that largely remains to be done with regard to psychosocial aspects of VDT use.

9

Design, Practice, and Standards for VDT Equipment and Work

Many video display terminals have been designed and introduced into workplaces with little attention to existing data and well-established principles of design and practice. There is a large base of knowledge about image quality, lighting and reflections, workplace design, and industrial and organizational psychology that has often been disregarded or inappropriately applied. It is likely that problems with and concerns about the comfort and performance of workers using VDTs would be greatly alleviated by the appropriate application of this knowledge to the design of VDT equipment and VDT jobs.

The first section of this chapter discusses specific ways in which this knowledge can be applied to enhance the comfort, performance, and job satisfaction of VDT workers. The second section examines guidelines and standards for VDT design that have been proposed or enacted into law in several European countries and Canada and discusses whether useful and appropriate standards should be established in the United States on the basis of present data.

PRINCIPLES OF GOOD DESIGN AND PRACTICE

Image Quality and Display Design

A number of display parameters that are known to influence visual performance (discussed in Chapter 4) may also influence operator comfort, but the relationships have not been quantitatively established. As a minimum, the following eight parameters should be considered in the design of displays:

1. Modulation transfer function (MTF) or other quality measures;

2. Acceptable color ranges (specified either as dominant wavelength and purity or as Commission Internationale de l'Eclairage [CIE] x,y coordinates);

3. Luminance and contrast for positive- and negative-contrast displays;

4. Dot-matrix and character sizes;

5. Character fonts;

6. Display jitter and geometric fidelity;

7. Specular and diffuse reflection coefficients; and

8. Number, spacing, and luminance profiles of video scan lines.

The use of existing data on visual processes and visual performance to determine appropriate values for these parameters could do much to prevent workplace problems. The complex considerations discussed in Chapter 4 preclude simply listing here a set or range of preferred values for these parameters. For many of them, compromises between ideal values and ergonomic and technological constraints are necessary; for others, existing data are not adequate to establish appropriate values, and further research is needed. Specific detailed procedures for measuring parameters of image quality should be established so that meaningful comparisons between VDT sets can be made.

Lighting and Reflections

The use of VDTs in workplaces in which the lighting is designed for traditional desk-top tasks is likely to adversely affect the comfort and performance of VDT operators. Virtually all of the problems associated with lighting and reflections in VDT workplaces can be eliminated or prevented by applying established principles of illuminating engineering, including lighting specification systems, in systematic workplace lighting design (discussed in Chapter 5).

Problems caused by inappropriate lighting can be classified into three general categories: (1) those caused by direct glare, (2) those caused by successive viewing of different luminances (transient adaptation), and (3) those caused by reflected glare and veiling reflections.

Minimizing Problems Caused by Direct Glare and Transient Adaptation

It is not possible to specify exact numerical values for lighting parameters for workplaces because of the enormous diversity of

VDT workplaces. We suggest that the values discussed in this section and in the references cited be treated as rough guidelines; a flexible approach is needed to optimize lighting conditions for particular tasks at particular workstations.

Discomfort glare and disability glare can be minimized in several ways (Stewart, 1980b; Christensen, 1981; Cole, 1981; see also Chapter 5). Direct glare problems caused by a bright light source, such as a window or luminaire, near a VDT screen can be solved simply by repositioning the screen; if repositioning is not possible, the light source should be screened. Workplace lighting should be designed so that the ratio of the luminance of the display to the luminance of the areas immediately surrounding the display is no higher than approximately 1:3. Areas not immediately surrounding the display but still within the operator's visual field should have luminances of approximately 5 to 10 times that of the display. Because the luminance of most displays is either fixed or can be adjusted only within a fairly narrow range, ambient illumination should be much lower than that typically used in offices; 300-500 lux of ambient illumination allows adequate visibility of both the display and hard-copy materials. It may be useful in some situations to lower ambient illumination still further; in this case it may be necessary to provide secondary lighting of hard-copy materials.

Measures that reduce direct glare also minimize the likelihood of problems with transient adaptation. In addition, the use of negative-contrast displays can reduce the likelihood of difficulty with transient adaptation. The use of negative-contrast displays does, however, involve some trade-offs and issues that are not yet resolved (see Chapters 4 and 5).

Minimizing Reflected Glare and Veiling Reflections

Several steps can be taken to minimize reflected glare and veiling reflections (Stewart, 1980b; Christensen, 1981; Cole, 1981; see also Chapter 5). Reflected glare from light sources such as windows and luminaires can be reduced by positioning the VDT screen perpendicular to the plane of the light sources. When such positioning is not possible, windows and luminaires should be shielded or screened: for example, parabolic wedge louvres can be used to reduce side light from luminaires. The use of VDTs in which the screen angle can be adjusted can also help in reducing reflections; a hood placed around the screen can help minimize veiling reflections.

Reflections off the front surface of a VDT screen can reduce the contrast and thus the visibility of the display image. Such reflections can also act as additional visual targets, which may promote fluctuations in accommodation and convergence. The use of negative-contrast displays may help to reduce these effects. The luminance of reflected images and thus their effect on the visibility of the display image can be reduced by reducing the reflectance of materials in the area surrounding the VDT. The luminance of reflected images can also be reduced by using filters of various types. While filters reduce the luminance of the reflected image with respect to the luminance of the display image, they also tend to diffuse the display image to varying degrees (see the discussion in Chapter 4).

Systematic Design of VDT Workstations

General Considerations

To achieve an ergonomically satisfactory workstation design, the multiple interactions between task, environment, and workplace elements must be considered (see the discussion in Chapter 6). The system components of the workstation include the display and its support, the keyboard and its support, the work seat, and the needed leg space in which foot controls may be located. All of these system elements are integrated through an operator, who determines system output and system dimensions.

A VDT must be located at the proper distance and elevation with respect to the human eye. The screen is usually located in front of the operator near the source document and possibly near the keyboard. Design parameters for the location of a VDT and its support are primarily determined by the operator's preferred viewing distance and preferred inclination of the line of sight (below the horizontal).

The same principal considerations apply to the source document (and its holder). Its distance from the operator is largely dependent on the operator's ability to focus clearly on the visual target, and its height depends on the operator's preferred inclination of the line of sight. These parameters are also influenced by the quality of illumination on the source document.

Manual work areas include the keyboard and writing surfaces. The keyboard itself should be detachable from the screen so that it can be located for the convenience and preference of the VDT operator. It therefore needs a separate support, adjustable independently of the screen support. While there is de facto agreement on the standard (QWERTY) keyboard with straight lines of keys arranged behind each other on a flat slope, current data indicate that other designs—such as a lateral tilt of separate left- and right-hand keyboards, including built-in wrist rests—may be preferable. Writing surfaces should be provided as needed, at an operator's preferred height and distance for ease of manipulation, support of the forearm, and convenience of seeing the target.

Leg room for a seated operator must provide ample space to accommodate variations in posture in the lower extremities, particularly knees and feet. Severe reductions in the height, width, or depth of leg room lead to confined postures that may be uncomfortable and unhealthful.

Hand, wrist, and arm supports are often said to be desirable, particularly for long-term periods of VDT operation, but there is little data on their presumed advantages. Guidelines have not yet been developed for support of hands and forearms.

The work seat is needed to support the body of a seated operator. While the seat pan carries most of the body weight, a properly designed backrest will also support some of the body weight. The main function of the backrest is to stabilize the body trunk and to provide suitable curvature of the spinal column. A high backrest with a properly incorporated neck support allows relaxation of neck and trunk muscles, particularly during work breaks. The backrest should be firmly attached to the seat pan and should have adjustable depth, height, and angle with respect to the seat pan. The seat pan itself should have a slight cavity in its center and should be well rounded along its front edge. Like the backrest, it should be firmly upholstered to evenly distribute the body weight.

A footrest is needed if the height adjustments of the supports for display, keyboard, and chair are not sufficiently variable to allow a comfortable posture for every operator who uses a given workstation. The footrest should have a large surface, and it should be slightly inclined with adjustable height.

The five-legged chair provides a more stable base with a shorter radius than the traditional four-legged chair; thus an operator's feet are kicked against the base less frequently. Overall, a five-legged chair seems to be more suitable than the four-legged chair and is now required in many European countries.

Specific Design and Use Guidelines

The following design guidelines apply primarily to a VDT workstation at which a person works many hours per day. As discussed in Chapter 6, this work situation probably imposes the most stringent requirements; if they are met, the workstation would also be suitable for occasional use.[1]

---

[1]Our design guidelines are largely derived from Ridder (1959); Kroemer (1970, 1971, 1981); Grandjean and Hunting, 1977;

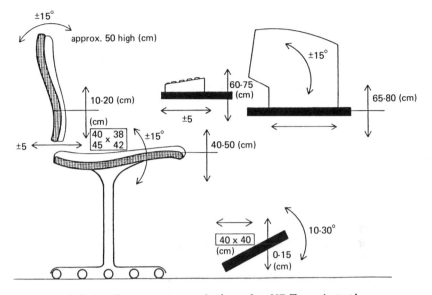

FIGURE 9.1 Design recommendations for VDT workstation components. SOURCE: Kroemer and Price (1982). Reprinted with permission of Industrial Engineering magazine, July, 1982. Copyright ⊛ Institute of Industrial Engineers, Inc., 25 Technology Park/Atlanta, Norcross, GA 30092.

The seat, keyboard, display, and foot support are interacting system components in the design of the workstation. Detailed design guidelines are shown in Figure 9.1, which gives suggested height ranges, angles, and other accommodations. The chair should be securely supported on four legs (or five casters as required in many European countries), and it should have adjustable seat pan and backrest heights. The angles of the seat pan and backrest should be adjustable relative to each other, and the backrest should also be adjustable front and back with respect to the seat pan.

In some situations the writing surface and the support surface

Grandjean (1980, 1981); Easterby et al., (1981); Grandjean and coworkers (1981); and National Institute for Occupational Safety and Health (1981). Van Cott and Kinkade (1972); Churchill et al. (1978); International Business Machines (1979); Cakir and coworkers (1980);Grandjean and Vigliani (1980); Mandal (1981); Olsen (1981); Rupp (1981); and Woodson (1981) summarize research results and present design recommendations.

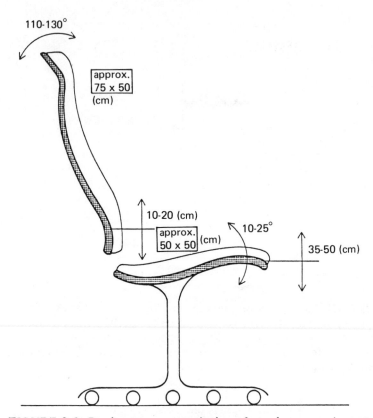

FIGURE 9.2 Design recommendations for a large work seat.

for the keyboard may need to be adjustable in height, front and back distance, and angulation. Finally, the footrest, if needed, may need to be adjustable in height, angulation, and front and back distance.

Figure 9.2 illustrates a chair that is larger than those usually used, with its dimensions increased in order to allow more flexibility in body position and support of upper back and neck. Several approaches may be taken to designing backrests that combine adequate support and mobility (see the discussion in Kroemer, 1983).

Job Design and Organizational Variables

There are a number of potential health-related outcomes associated with psychosocial stressors that may occur with improper

VDT use. Lack of control, low social support, heavy (quantitative) workload, and underutilization of skills and abilities can all occur within the context of VDT-related tasks (see Chapter 8). The literature we reviewed indicates that these stressors can affect mental and physical states.

Variation in the Task and Task Environment

There are a number of strategies for reducing workers' strain. Two of them are job rotation and rest breaks, to allow variety in the work and recovery from intense exposure to psychosocial stressors. With regard to work breaks, the National Institute for Occupational Safety and Health (1981:70) has recommended that

1. A 15-minute work-rest break should be taken after two hours of continuous VDT work for operators under moderate visual demands and/or moderate workload.

2. A 15-minute work-rest break should be taken after one hour of continuous VDT work for operators under high visual demands, high workload and/or those engaged in repetitive work tasks.

We note, however, that "moderate" and "high" visual demands and workloads are not defined by NIOSH, and no comparison is made between VDT jobs and comparable non-VDT jobs on these parameters.

A report issued by the Department of Health of New Zealand (Coe et al., 1980) finds that although fatiguelike complaints about the eyes are not alleviated by mandated formal breaks, they are alleviated by informal breaks, that is, time spent not viewing the screen, which may include time spent performing other work tasks. These findings support two major principles in Chapter 8: (1) low stress can be thought of as the goodness of fit between individuals and their environment, rather than the standardization of environments regardless of individual needs and abilities; and (2) participation in decision making or some degree of individual control over the nature and pace of the work allows people to exercise maximum person-environment fit because each person is assumed to be the best judge of the needs for rest breaks. The recommendation of a fixed rest break is not supported by those principles. (The NIOSH recommendations need to be reconciled with such findings.) One can imagine instances in which an imposed rest break might prove very strain-producing for an operator who is highly involved in a task and who wants to finish the task without interruption.

If rest breaks should be flexible, are there any other principles that should govern them? In the 1920s and 1930s much of the research in industrial psychology was directed toward finding optimal placement and duration of rest periods; the research was summarized in the first edition of the text by Ghiselli and Brown (1948:249):

1. Rest should be introduced when performance is at a maximum, just before a reduction in productivity. The timing of rest is more important than the length of the rest period, although optimal rest period lengths can also be determined for individual jobs.

2. Rest periods may be more useful for relatively ineffective workers; better workers seem to develop more efficient procedures and therefore have less need for rest. [It would be valuable to know whether this finding applies to performance of near-visual work, a question not asked in this early research.]

3. Rest periods are most effective with work requiring concentration than on jobs that are more or less automatic and leave the employee free to daydream, converse with others, or follow similar monotony reducing strategies.

In the many years since most of the research was done, rest periods have been determined more by negotiation than by empirical research. However, it would again be useful to determine, independently for data entry or for more screen-intensive work, the curves showing productivity, performance decrements, and optimal rest period timing to attempt to relieve visual discomfort.

Other Strategies for Good Employee Management

Another strategy for reducing workers' strain is allowing a VDT user the authority to delegate workload under conditions of overload or to pace the input of workload according to his or her tolerances. Supervisors can also be trained to seek feedback on the input, production, and output of work (Katz and Kahn, 1978) so that work can be allocated according to a worker's ability to process it. Reward systems can be instituted that provide a supervisor with incentives for promoting workers' well-being, low turnover, and low absenteeism, as well as for promoting high productivity. Similarly, reward systems can be instituted that provide VDT users with incentives to give feedback when they experience excessive strain and when they perceive poor person-environment fit.

General principles of employee participation should be used to maximize the quality of strain-reducing strategies and adherence to them (Vroom and Yetton [1973] discuss decision points in determining whether participation is appropriate). Otherwise, even well-intentioned changes in work procedures, such as job rotation, delegation of work to others, and feedback to supervisors may be resisted both because employees want to maintain a sense of control and because they perceive genuine penalties in adopting the changes. For example, it is unlikely that feedback to supervisors about excessive workload can be unilaterally mandated: with only a simple mandate from management, an experienced worker may wisely decide that exercising the feedback option could threaten a possible future pay increase.

It is obviously difficult to make specific suggestions about employee management for all possible VDT work situations in which such advice might be applied. In general, humane management techniques should be applied to the design of VDT work as they should for any other type of work. There is a large body of knowledge in industrial and organizational psychology on the determinants of employee satisfaction (see, e.g., Katzell and Yankelovich, 1975; Kahn, 1981).[2] An organization planning to integrate VDT-related technology into the larger design of jobs should examine some of the suggestions that derive from that literature. We also suggest that organizations that are making a major commitment to VDT technology consider initiating their own investigations of the psychosocial components of the job design. In this way, organizations can supplement the existing knowledge regarding psychosocial stressors and their relation to the use of VDTs. If organizations do undertake such research, they could make significant advances in knowledge by adopting research designs that are specifically intended to test causal models over time and are intended to evaluate simultaneously several competing explanations for hypothesized health outcomes (for detailed discussions of such designs, see, e.g., Cooke and Campbell, 1976; Joreskog and Sorbom, 1979; Kenny, 1979).

---

[2]Katzell and Yankelovich (1975) summarize research that shows that the basic conditions of good working circumstances for both an employee's emotional well-being and high productivity include competent supervision, fair pay, job security, good working conditions with regard to the physical parameters of work and the fit between the nature of the work and the person's needs and abilities, and good relationships with employers and employer representatives.

STANDARDS AND GUIDELINES FOR VDT DESIGN[3]

Standards that specify values for various workstation and workplace design parameters have been enacted or proposed in several countries. Individual and group-authored papers in the technical literature have also recommended guideline values for various parameters. Several of the more widely known guidelines and standards are summarized in Tables 9.1-9.8. There is considerable disagreement in the specifications of some design parameters in these guidelines and standards (see Brown et al., 1982), and some authors have criticized some standards as inappropriate or untimely (see, e.g., Rupp, 1981).

The various guidelines and standards differ considerably in their underlying assumptions. Some specifications are oriented toward issues of performance; others are more concerned with issues of comfort. Because the relationship between comfort and performance is unknown for most tasks (but is likely to be complex) and because comfort and performance are not necessarily positively correlated, recommended specifications differ among various guidelines and standards. Research is needed to establish the relationships between comfort and performance in VDT-related work; such research would assist efforts to develop guidelines for the design of VDTs that take account of both factors.

The various specifications may also conflict because some guidelines and standards include considerations of interactions between variables and others do not. For example, few of the standards take into account the well-established and quantified interaction between contrast and character size in determining character legibility. Another reason for conflicting specifications is that research on requirements for VDTs in office use is a relatively new research area, and the best approaches have yet to be established. (Some researchers who have been active in other areas have turned their attention to needs in this area without becoming adept at human performance research in VDT applica-

---

[3]We use <u>standards</u> to refer to specifications of values for design parameters to which strict adherence is expected. The term includes legally binding specifications, such as the German Safety Standards; specifications written into contracts, such as the U.S. Military Standards 1472B and 1472C; and specifications voluntarily adopted by industry, such as those promulgated by the American National Standards Institute. In contrast, we use <u>guidelines</u> to refer to specifications that are suggested with the understanding that implementation be flexible, depending on circumstances and needs.

TABLE 9.1 Recommended Key Characteristics for VDTs

Source	Size	Spacing	Travel	Force	Feedback
Canadian DCIEM (Gorrell, 1980)	Concave[a]				
Groupe de Recherche sur les Ecrans Visuelisation (Rey and Meyer, 1977)					
German DIN Standard 66234 (Deutsche Institut für Normungen, 1982)					
German Safety Standards (Zentralstelle für Unfallverhütung und Arbeitsmedizin, 1980)					
Snyder and Maddox (1978)					
Swedish National Board of Occupational Safety and Health (1979)					
Technical University of Berlin (Cakir et al., 1978)	13 mm	20 mm center-to-center	5-8 mm	0.26-1.5 N	tactile preferred, acoustic
University of London (Reading, 1978)					
MIL STD 1472B (U.S. Department of Defense, 1974)[b]	10-14 mm; 13 mm preferred	≤ 6.4 mm edge-to-edge	0.8-4.8 mm numeric; 1.3-6.3 mm alphanumeric	1-4 N; 0.25-1.5 N preferred	
Video Display Terminals (Cakir et al, 1980)	12-15 mm	18-20 mm center-to-center	0.8-8 mm	0.25-1.5 N	acoustic, tactile, or snap action

[a] No size specified; should be concave shape.
[b] See MIL STD 1472C (U.S. Department of Defense, 1981) for additional information.

TABLE 9.2 Recommended Keyboard Characteristics for VDTs

Source	Height	Slope	Thickness	Detachment
Canadian DCIEM (Gorrell, 1980)				
Groupe de Recherche sur les Ecrans Visuelisation (Rey and Meyer, 1977)				
German DIN Standard 66234 (Deutsche Institut für Normungen, 1982)	≤ 30 mm above table top		≤ 30 mm; otherwise recessed	Preferred for clerical work
German Safety Standards (Zentralstelle für Unfallverhütung und Arbeitsmedizin, 1980)	≤ 30 mm above table top	≤ 15°	Palm rest if > 30 mm	Required except for unique applications
Snyder and Maddox (1978)				
Swedish National Board of Occupational Safety and Health (1979)				
Technical University of Berlin (Cakir et al., 1978)	≤ 75 cm above floor	≤ 5°	≤ 30 mm; otherwise recessed	Preferred
University of London (Reading, 1978)				
MIL STD 1472B (U.S. Department of Defense, 1974)[a]		15-25°; 16-17° preferred		
Video Display Terminals (Cakir et al., 1980)	≤ 50 mm above table top; 30 mm preferred	5-15°; palm rest	≤ 50 mm; 30 mm preferred	

[a] See MIL STD 1472C (U.S. Department of Defense, 1981) for additional information.

TABLE 9.3   Recommended Display Spacing for VDTs

Source	Character Format	Line Spacing	Column Spacing	Display Size
Canadian DCIEM (Gorrell, 1980)	≥ 5 × 7			16 rows of 64 characters, minimum
Groupe de Recherche sur les Ecrans Visuelisation (Rey and Meyer, 1977)				
German DIN Standard 66234 (Deutsche Institut für Normungen, 1982)	≥ 5 × 7	1 dot or 10% character height	1 dot or 10% character height "Not touch each other"	
German Safety Standards (Zentralstelle für Unfallverhütung und Arbeitsmedizin, 1980)	clear and unambiguous			Adequate amount of information
Snyder and Maddox (1978)	≥ 5 × 7; 7 × 9 Huddleston or Lincoln/Mitre preferred			
Swedish National Board of Occupational Safety and Health (1979)				
Technical University of Berlin (Cakir et al., 1978)	Vertical	100-500% character height	50% character width	
University of London (Reading, 1978)	≥ 5 × 7 to 12 × 18	character height	50% character width	
MIL STD 1472B (U.S. Department of Defense, 1974)[a]				
Video Display Terminals (Cakir et al., 1980)	≥ 5 × 7; > 7 × 9 preferred	100-150% character height	20-50% character height	

[a] See MIL STD 1472C (U.S. Department of Defense, 1981) for additional information.

TABLE 9.4 Recommended Symbol Characteristics for VDTs

Source	Luminance[a]	Contrast[b]	Size	Percent Active Area
Canadian DCIEM (Gorrell, 1980) Groupe de Recherche sur les Ecrans Visuelisation (Rey and Meyer, 1977)	85 cd/m²	≥ 4:1	≥ 3.5 mm	75
German DIN Standard 66234 (Deutsche Institut für Normungen, 1982)		3:1 to 15:1; 6:1 to 10:1 preferred	≥ 18 arcmin; 2.6 mm preferred	
German Safety Standards (Zentralstelle für Unfallverhütung und Arbeitsmedizin, 1980)		3:1 to 15:1; 6:1 to 10:1 preferred	≥ 18 arcmin	
Snyder and Maddox (1978)	65 cd/m²	≥ 3:1; > 15:1 preferred	15-21 arcmin	No visible structure
Swedish National Board of Occupational Safety and Health (1979)				No visible structure
Technical University of Berlin (Cakir et al., 1978)		5:1 to 10:1	≥ 16 arcmin; 20 arcmin preferred 15.2-20.6 arcmin	
University of London (Reading, 1978) MIL STD 1472B (U.S. Department of Defense, 1974)[c]		4:1	≥ 20 arcmin and 10 lines for CRT; ≥ 15 arcmin for others	
Video Display Terminals (Cakir et al., 1980)	45 cd/m² minimum; 80-160 cd/m² preferred	≥ 3:1; 8:1-10:1 optimum	15-20 arcmin or 3.1-4.2 mm	

[a] 3.426 cd/m² = 1 ft-L.
[b] Assumes positive contrast.
[c] See MIL STD 1472C (U.S. Department of Defense, 1981) for additional information.

TABLE 9.5 Recommended Screen Characterstics for VDTs

Source	Preferred Color	Phosphor	Contrast[a]	Refresh Rate
Canadian DCIEM (Gorrell, 1980)	Green or white	Short persistence		60/60[b]
Groupe de Recherche sur les Ecrans Visuelisation (Rey and Meyer, 1977)	Not red		Negative preferred	
German DIN Standard 66234 (Deutsche Institut für Normungen, 1982)	Green through orange			25 frames per second/ 50 Hz for positive; higher for negative
German Safety Standards (Zentralstelle für Unfallverhütung und Arbeitsmedizin, 1980) Snyder and Maddox (1978) Swedish National Board of Occupational Safety and Health (1979)	Not red or blue		Negative preferred	Flicker-free
Technical University of Berlin (Cakir et al., 1978)	Yellow-green	P4, P31	Negative preferred	Flicker-free (50 Hz)
University of London (Reading, 1978)		Medium persistence		25/50 or 30/60[b]
MIL STD 1472B (U.S. Department of Defense, 1974)[c]			Either for high illumination; positive for low	
Video Display Terminals (Cakir et al., 1980)	Personal preference	P4, P31		25/50 or 30/60[b]

[a] Negative contrast is dark on light, equals positive polarity.
[b] Frames per second/fields per second.
[c] See MIL STD 1472C (U.S. Department of Defense, 1981) for additional information.

TABLE 9.6   Recommended Illumination and Glare Characteristics for VDTs

Source	Illumination[a]	Glare Control
Canadian DCIEM (Gorrell, 1980)	807-1076 lux	Antireflection treatment required
Groupe de Recherche sur les Ecrans Visuelisation (Rey and Meyer, 1977)		
German DIN Standard 66234 (Deutsche Institut für Normungen, 1982)	300-500 lux for positive contrast; ≥ 500 lux for negative contrast	Diffusing surface, micromesh filters, optical coatings, sprays, hoods, combination filters
German Safety Standards (Zentralstelle für Unfallverhütung und Arbeitsmedizin, 1980)		Avoid disturbing reflections
Snyder and Maddox (1978)	≤ 75 lux	Antireflection treatment as needed to obtain contrast required
Swedish National Board of Occupational Safety and Health (1979)	200-300 lux; supplement as required	Avoid bright reflections
Technical University of Berlin (Cakir et al., 1978)	500 lux	Avoid focusable reflections; diffusing surface
University of London (Reading, 1978)	500-750 lux	Avoid reflections that reduce information transfer
MIL STD 1472B (U.S. Department of Defense, 1974)[b]	≥ 540 lux; 1075 lux preferred; consistent with other tasks	
Video Display Terminals (Cakir et al., 1980)	300-500 lux	Optical coating, diffusing surface, polarization filter, micromesh filter

[a] 10.76 lux = 1 ft-candle.
[b] See MIL STD 1472C (U.S. Department of Defense, 1981) for additional information.

TABLE 9.7 Viewing Geometry Recommendations for VDTs

Source	Viewing Distance	Tilt Angle	Display Height	Image Distortion
Canadian DCIEM (Gorrell, 1980)		Normal ± 5° to line of sight	Center 10-20° below horizon	
Groupe de Recherche sur les Ecrans Visuelisation (Rey and Meyer, 1977)				
German DIN Standard 66234 (Deutsche Institut für Normungen, 1982)	50-70 cm	≤ 5° down, ≤ 20° up	Top at 37-52 mm above table surface	≤ 2% of width, ≤ 10% character size
German Safety Standards (Zentralstelle für Unfallverhütung und Arbeitsmedizin, 1980)			Top below horizon; center at 35° preferred	Not impair legibility
Snyder and Maddox (1978)	Not critical; optimize angular subtense			
Swedish National Board of Occupational Safety and Health (1979)	Individually adjustable	Adjustable		
Technical University of Berlin (Carkin et al., 1978)	50 cm	None, vertical	Below eye height, 20° below horizon	
University of London (Reading, 1978)	≤ 2/3 of accommodation range			
MIL STD 1472B (U.S. Department of Defense, 1974)[a] *Video Display Terminals* (Cakir et al., 1980)	≤ 70 cm	Normal ± 45° to line of sight Adjustable	150 to 1200 mm above seat Top below horizon	

[a] See MIL STD 1472C (U.S. Department of Defense, 1981) for additional information.

TABLE 9.8   Recommended Workstation Dimensions for VDTs (mm)

Source	Work Surface			Knee Room		
	Height	Width	Depth	Height	Width	Depth
Canadian DCIEM (Gorrell, 1980)						
Groupe de Recherche sur les Ecrans Visuelisation (Rey and Meyer, 1977)						
German DIN Standard 66234 (Deutsche Institut für Normungen, 1982)	650-750; ≤720 if fixed	≥1200	900	≥660; 690 preferred	≥1200	
German Safety Standards (Zentralstelle für Unfallverhütung und Arbeitsmedizin, 1980)	680-760; 720 if fixed	≥1200; 1600 preferred	50-100 in front of keys	≥650; 690 preferred	580	600
Snyder and Maddox (1978)						
Swedish National Board of Occupational Safety and Health (1979)						
Technical University of Berlin (Cakir et al., 1978)	650-750; 720 if fixed			690		
University of London (Reading, 1978)						
MIL STD 1472B (U.S. Department of Defense, 1974)[a]	740-790	≥760	≥400	≥640	≥510	≥460
Video Display Terminals (Cakir et al., 1980)	≤720				800	700

[a] See MIL STD 1472C (U.S. Department of Defense, 1981) for additional information.

tions; this is another factor in conflicting specifications among various guidelines and standards.) Examples of topics on which further study is needed are image characteristics, keyboard height, and needs for wristrests.

Because there are many types of VDT applications, the number and variety of applications are growing rapidly, and there are major differences in VDT workstation operations, different guidelines or standards are likely to be required for significantly different applications and operations. Simplified specifications or guidelines can be misleading and seductively comforting. Blind compliance with guidelines or attemping to purchase a VDT for use for any task under any circumstances can lead to obvious difficulties. Both research and careful deliberation will be required to deal with the heterogeneity of applications.

In this situation, we believe it is too early to establish mandatory standards. In particular there is a danger that rigid standards would stifle technological improvements and new approaches. Thus we recommend that the United States not now attempt to establish mandatory standards for VDT design. Rather, we urge three concurrent courses of action. First, users and manufacturers should become familiar with the technical literature in this area and solicit the advice and assistance of knowledgeable professionals in the design and installation of VDT equipment and the layout of workstations. Second, there should be continued dialogue between scientists, manufacturers, and users in efforts to evolve guidelines and minimum standards appropriate to particular applications. Third, research should be directed at unresolved questions about the effects of display and workstation parameters on worker comfort and performance. At the same time, judicious use of guidelines to suggest reasonable values for design parameters is useful and desirable.

10
Research Needs

In the preceding chapters we have emphasized our conclusion that application of existing knowledge would reduce the incidence of complaints and symptoms of job-related ocular and musculo-skeletal discomfort and stress reported by VDT workers. In addition, however, a number of questions raised in our analysis of the research literature on effects of VDT work remain unanswered and merit attention. Many of these questions could be answered by appropriately designed research, and in this chapter we suggest several lines of research that might be useful. However, we urge that competing priorities in the field of occupational health be carefully considered before undertaking research on VDT work.

EFFECTS OF DISPLAYS ON VISUAL ACTIVITY

Objective Correlates of Visual Complaints

A programmatic research effort should be oriented toward relating objective measures of visual activity to subjective complaints of ocular discomfort and visual difficulties. Much of the difficulty in conducting or evaluating such research stems from the poor definition of "visual fatigue" and the lack of established correlations among measures of ocular discomfort, visual performance, and physiological variables. Studies should be conducted to measure visual functions, such as eye movements (e.g., frequency and duration of fixations and saccades, scan patterns) and changes in pupil size and accommodation, and to relate these measures to visual symptoms reported by subjects. Since eye-movement patterns have been related to display quality by several research efforts, it seems logical that measures of visual activity

214

could be related to subjective symptoms in a realistic working environment. The displays used in this research should be systematically varied, from those that are considered to be of poor quality to those that are considered to be of good quality. Useful optical measures of image quality have been defined by several investigators (see Chapter 4).

It is extremely important that such research be conducted using longitudinal designs and that workers should be studied while spending considerable time performing meaningful, realistic tasks that might induce visual symptoms. Brief laboratory studies of the type often used in research on visual performance are not adequate to address questions in this area. With this approach it should be possible to relate the quality of a displayed image to measurements of visual functions and to such subjective symptoms as ocular discomfort.

Relating Display Characteristics to Workplace Conditions

Research is needed to relate display design characteristics to workplace illumination and the effective suppression of glare. After first doing everything possible in the workplace to eliminate sources of direct and indirect glare or to reduce their effects, two further approaches to suppressing glare should be studied: use of glare-reduction filters and changes in display image polarity.

The effectiveness of filters should be measured as a function of environmental parameters, such as types of glare and location of glare sources. The effects of various types of filters on image quality and contrast transmission should be measured to determine whether visual task performance is actually improved by a given filter type in a given environment. This research is critically needed to cut through the morass of arbitrary, capricious, and often misleading claims made by some filter manufacturers.

Careful research is needed to compare the effects of positive- and negative-contrast displays on visual task performance and visual symptoms. Because a negative-contrast display probably requires different refresh rates, different stroke widths, and different contrast ratios than does a positive-contrast display, a moderately large investment would be necessary to achieve the equipment control required for this research. Once the control over such equipment is obtained, however, the research could be conducted in the same environment used to measure visual activity, visual performance, and subjective estimates of discomfort, as described above.

Effects of Image Instability

Research is needed on the possible effects on visual function caused by geometric and positional instability of display images. The frame-to-frame jitter of a CRT image, however small, may cause visual difficulties, especially during prolonged viewing. Comparisons between representative CRT displays and geometrically stable (e.g., flat-panel) displays would permit an evaluation of possible effects. Here, too, research should be conducted using realistic task conditions and long enough viewing times to induce symptoms.

Distinguishing Specific Effects of VDTs

Visual complaints and symptoms should be examined as a function of work time for various segments of the working population. Work is inherently tiring, and visual work may be inherently visually tiring. Thus, it is important that the time course of visual complaints and symptoms be accurately measured for a variety of displays, to distinguish the effects of visual work from the effects of visual displays per se. This research should use various representative segments of workers, including those with good and those with poor eyesight and younger as well as older workers.

PSYCHOSOCIAL STRESSORS

Our review of the published literature on psychosocial stressors in VDT work reveals many questions that have not been adequately addressed: How should VDT work be characterized and how could its characteristics be reliably measured? What psychosocial variables of work should be measured in VDT studies? What physical conditions of work settings need to be measured and controlled in the study of psychosocial stressors in VDT use? Does the amount or kind of VDT use increase or decrease some psychosocial stressors, such as isolation from others? What parameters of rest periods (e.g., duration, frequency, spacing, flexibility) should be studied in relation to worker well-being? To what extent is well-being influenced by the manner in which VDT technology is introduced into the workplace?

We caution, however, that the payoff for research on questions about psychosocial stressors unique to VDT work seems likely to be low. Given the flaws in existing studies, it cannot be determined whether most of the differences reported between VDT work and non-VDT work are attributable to the use of VDT technology per se. Aspects of work such as workload, social support, and task complexity that are not specific to VDT work have been confounded with aspects such as display design that are specific. The nonspecific aspects have clearer empirical links to mental and physical well-being than does the use of VDTs. Consequently, we suggest that higher priority be given to studies of parameters such as workload, social support, and task complexity that affect all jobs, not just those involving VDTs.

Appendix A

A Review of Methodology in Studies of Visual Functions During VDT Tasks

John O. Merritt

This appendix reviews field and laboratory studies of temporary changes in various oculomotor functions in subjects during the course of performing VDT tasks for a period of up to several hours. Only a few such studies have been published; this review discusses the four studies that constitute virtually the entire literature in this area as of mid-1982. The one known exception is a study by Murch (1982b) that measured changes in visual function in subjects performing tasks at two different types of VDTs; it is not included here because insufficient detail for a review was provided in the brief published report.

One study reviewed here also compared changes in measures of visual function in subjects performing VDT and hard-copy tasks. Although the changes in visual function reported in these studies were interpreted by the investigators as evidence of "visual fatigue" associated with viewing VDTs, this interpretation is uncertain. Two of the studies reviewed here included questionnaires regarding symptoms of ocular discomfort. Although the investigators concluded that symptoms of ocular discomfort are associated with changes in visual function, they did not report whether the variables were statistically related.

There are, of course, many practical difficulties in designing and conducting this kind of research. This review is intended to provide an illustration of the kinds of difficulties encountered.

John O. Merritt, who is a senior scientist with Perceptronics, Inc., was a consultant to the panel. The author gratefully acknowledges the opportunity to review a prepublication copy of a critique of human factors research on VDTs (Helander et al., 1983).

Gunnarsson, E., and Soderberg, I. 1980. Eyestrain Resulting from VDT Work at the Swedish Telecommunications
Administration. Eye Changes and Visual Strain During
Various Working Procedures. Stockholm: National Board
of Occupational Safety and Health.

Gunnarsson and Soderberg measured changes in the near points of
accommodation and convergence under normal and intensified
conditions of VDT use. Questionnaires and interviews were also
used to obtain information regarding symptoms of "visual strain."
The report argues that changes in the near point of convergence
may be a useful objective measure of visual strain associated with
VDT work.

The measures of accommodative and convergence near points
were based on subjective responses. The authors report that
changes in both near points were greater under intensified than
under normal conditions, but the data are given only in the form of
graphs; the statistical analyses performed are not described, and
the level of significance is not stated. The data are presented
only as mean values of changes; absolute levels and variances in
the data are not reported. Because of the recriprocal nature of
optical power measures, a change in the near point of accommodation—for example, from 10 to 13 cm—represents a far
greater loss in accommodation than a change from 20 to 23 cm.

The subjects were self-selected samples of opportunity; no
comparison or control group of subjects performing non-VDT work
was used. The authors did not report whether normal and intensified conditions were counterbalanced. No attempt was made to
determine if task variables and subjective responses regarding
symptoms of visual strain were statistically related to the
measured changes in optometric functions.

Haider, M., Kundi, M., and Weissenbock, M. 1980. Worker
strain related to VDUs with differently coloured characters. Pp. 53-64 in E. Grandjean and E. Vigliani, eds.,
Ergonomic Aspects of Visual Display Terminals. London:
Taylor & Francis.

Haider and coworkers measured visual acuity in 13 VDT operators
and a comparison group of 9 non-VDT workers before and after
four 3-hour sessions. Subjective state, chromatic adaptation,
degree of optical illusion, subjective visual acuity, subjective color
vision, and heart rate were also measured. A questionnaire on
asthenopia and other physical symptoms was administered
following the test sessions. No details are presented, but apparently the relationship between reported physical symptoms and

visual acuity was not assessed. Each subject in the VDT group was tested for two of the sessions using a VDT with green characters and for the other two sessions using a VDT with yellow characters. The VDT group performed a test protocol; the non-VDT group performed their normal office work (primarily typing). The authors reported that a statistically significant temporary reduction in visual acuity occurred following the test sessions in the VDT group, while the comparison group showed almost no change in acuity. The reduction in acuity was greater when VDTs having green characters were used. The authors referred to the temporary reduction in acuity as "temporary myopization" and attributed it to "accommodation strain."

Several aspects of the design of this study and the analysis of results make this interpretation uncertain. The data are presented in the form of graphs; absolute values are not reported, the statistical analyses performed are not described, and although changes in acuity for the VDT group are reported to be statistically significant, the level of significance is not reported.

Visual acuity was measured using wall charts at a distance of 4 m; accommodation was not measured. This method is subject to influences resulting from factors other than changes in accommodation caused by temporary myopic defocus blur. For example, general fatigue (which has been shown to be associated with pupillary constriction and a resulting reduction in the need for accommodation—see the discussion in Chapter 7) following the 3-hour test session could have affected the measurements, either through its effect on pupil size or by influencing the motivation of the subjects. It is also possible that spatial frequency adaptation to the VDT and source documents could have reduced contrast sensitivity to the letters and numerals of the wall chart, reducing measured acuity.

The comparison group, which showed almost no change in visual acuity following work, consisted of non-VDT workers performing traditional office work, mainly typing. Because the tasks performed by this group were quite different from the test protocol performed by the VDT group and because subjects in the two groups were not appropriately matched in other respects, no conclusions can be drawn regarding the relative effects of VDT and hard-copy displays on visual acuity.

The approach taken in the comparison of acuity changes between subjects using VDTs having green or yellow characters is promising, since it recognizes that the particular type of VDT display used may make a difference in the kinds of optometric effects that could be associated with prolonged or intensive use. The study also attempted to obtain test-retest measures by using two different green and two different yellow VDTs in a within-subjects design with an appropriately counterbalanced order.

Unfortunately, the authors did not provide sufficient detail for evaluation of their measurement apparatus and methods, the distribution of acuity values for each of their 13 VDT subjects for each of the four test sessions, and the inherent variability of their measures over time.

Although absolute values are not reported, the graphs indicate that the mean acuity decrement associated with VDTs having yellow characters was approximately 0.14 diopter; the decrement for VDTs having green characters was approximtely 0.24 diopter. The postwork acuities correspond to approximately 20/21 for the yellow and 20/24 for the green. All else being equal, yellow characters would require more accommodative effort than green characters; the finding that yellow character displays produced less "temporary myopization" suggests that accommodative effort may not be related in a simple way to decrements in acuity.

The small decrements in acuity reported in this study are typically found following a wide variety of visually demanding tasks that do not involve VDTs (see Chapter 7) and thus would not represent a deterioration of visual function specific to VDTs.

Mourant, R. R., Lakshmanan, R., and Chantadisal, R. 1981. Visual fatigue and cathode ray tube display terminals. Human Factors 23(5): 529-540.

Mourant and coworkers measured the length of time taken during a visual search and reading task to focus from a near point to a far point (termed outfocus time) and back again on the near point (termed infocus time) as a function of display type (CRT or hard copy) at the near point, subjects' age, and time on task. (Only the authors' Study II is considered here; Study I, which used only two subjects, is not discussed for that reason.) The study reports that outfocus time and infocus time were significantly higher for the CRT display and that both times increased as a function of time on task for both the CRT display and the hard-copy display. Neither outfocus nor infocus times differed significantly as a function of age. These results are interpreted as evidence of fatigue in eye movement, or accommodative mechanisms, or both.

Several aspects of the design of this study are either unspecified, or if specified, are problematic in the analysis of the results. For example, the viewing distances from the subjects to the CRT or hard copy are not specified, and whether these distances were controlled is not reported. The visual angles subtended by the near and far targets are also not reported, despite the importance of these factors in accommodative response. Information on relative characteristics of the CRT, hard-copy, and distant target displays--for example, polarity and character sizes--is not presented, even though these characteristics affect the accommodative response required for the tasks given.

The method used to determine outfocus and infocus times was subjective analysis of videotapes of the subjects as they alternately searched a near target (distance from the subject not specified) and performed a reading task on a far target (6 m from the subject). The indicators used to delineate outfocus and infocus times are not clearly described. Thus it is not possible to determine, for example, how accurately the outfocus time was discriminated in the analysis of the videotapes from the read time on the distant target or how accurately the infocus and search times were discriminated on the near target. Data on the performance of the subjects, which might be expected to be related to outfocus and infocus times, are not reported. In view of the subjective nature and inherent variability and imprecision of this type of measure, there may be no practical significance in the small differences in mean outfocus and infocus times for the CRT display compared with the hard-copy display (mean outfocus time of 0.013 seconds longer and mean infocus time of 0.012 seconds longer for the CRT), and the increase in outfocus and infocus times for both displays as a function of time on task may have no practical significance. An additional limitation on this type of measurement is that the time taken to perform the viewing sequence is dependent on the motivation and level of general fatigue of the subject, independent of the study's hypothesized fatigue of the ocular muscles.

It is known that the latency of accommodation and the rate at which it can be changed vary between subjects and also for the same subject under different conditions (see Chapter 7); however, no attempt is reported to obtain data on the normal variability of accommodative response in the subjects. It is possible that small changes such as those reported may be due to this normal variability. In addition, although the distance to the near target was not specified, it is assumed to be approximately 20 inches (normal reading distance); thus, both near and far targets could have simultaneously been within the subjects' depth of focus, requiring no difference in accommodation.

Although the findings are reported as statistically significant, the statistical analyses performed are not clearly described. Outfocus and infocus times are likely to be highly correlated, but it appears that a multivariate analysis was not performed and that various possible interactions among variables were not examined. For example, although the purpose of this study was to compare accommodative response to CRT and paper displays, the data on relative increases during performance of the task in outfocus and infocus times for the two types of display are not reported. Thus it is not possible to determine whether the small differences in outfocus and infocus times between the CRT display condition and the hard-copy condition were constant from the beginning of the experiment (i.e., no interaction between type of display and time on the task) or whether, as the study concludes, "a larger increase occurred during the CRT task than in the hard-copy search."

The small number of subjects (six) used in this study makes it difficult to generalize the results. In addition, four of the subjects were older than 50 years and thus presumably had little or no accommodation. Consequently, it is unlikely that accommodation played a significant role in the results; the fact that neither outfocus nor infocus times varied as a function of age supports the idea that accommodation was problably not a significant factor.

The attempt in this study to compare CRT and hard-copy tasks is a potentially valuable approach; however, because of problems in methodology and analysis, the conclusion that use of a CRT for 2 to 3 hours has a "measurable fatigue impact on the visual mechanism and that impact is greater for CRT viewing than for hard-copy viewing" does not seem warranted. In addition, the conclusion seems to be based on the assumption that changes in measures of optometric functions signify changes in the level of fatigue of ocular muscles; this assumption has not been scientifically established as fact.

Östberg, O. 1980. Accommodation and visual fatigue in display work. Pp. 41-52 in E. Grandjean and E. Vigliani, eds., Ergonomic Aspects of Visual Display Terminals. London: Taylor & Francis.

Östberg compared dark focus (measured with a target at 6 m) and accommodative response to targets at distances varying from 0.25 m to 1 m for three groups of subjects: air traffic controllers, telephone sales clerks performing a mixture of VDT and traditional office work, and telephone directory operators performing continuous VDT work. No control groups of workers performing comparable non-VDT work were included. Measurements were made before and after VDT work, using a laser optometer. Östberg reported a statistically significant shift in the mean dark focus of the air traffic controllers from 0.94 diopter before work to 1.62 diopters following work; the air traffic controllers were also reported to show statistically significant reduced accommodative responses following work, becoming more myopic for distant targets and more hyperopic for near targets. Absolute values of changes in accommodative response were not reported; however, examination of the graphs indicates that the values were fairly small. Changes in dark focus and accommodative response also occurred in the other two groups, but these changes were reported as not statistically significant.

Although Östberg attributed the findings for the air traffic controllers to their visually demanding VDT work, and refers to the changes in optometric function as evidence of visual fatigue associated with VDT work, several aspects of the design of the study make these interpretations uncertain. (The term visual fatigue apparently was used in this study to refer to accommodative state rather than to visual discomfort, which apparently was not assessed.)

The display screen used by the air traffic controllers was located at a distance of 65 cm from the subjects, requiring only 1.5 diopters of accommodation. This value approximates the dark focus for many individuals (Leibowitz and Owens, 1978) and thus should not require unusual accommodative effort; it is also similar to the reported mean dark focus of the air traffic controllers measured following work (1.62 diopters).

The ambient working environment for the air traffic controllers was not described, but it can be assumed that the level of ambient illumination was low, which is typical of air traffic control workplaces. The reduction in accommodative response following work may have been caused by pupillary constriction resulting from the shift from subdued lighting conditions during work to the 250 cd/m^2 luminance (reported in an earlier publication on the results for the air traffic controllers by Östberg et al. [1980]) of the test cards used in the vision tests following work. Although pupil diameter was not measured in this study, it is known that pupillary constriction increases the depth of focus of the eye and thus reduces the need for accommodation; in addition, pupillary constriction influences accommodation directly (see Chapter 7). Pupillary constriction and thus a reduction in the amplitude of accommodation is also known to occur in subjects who are fatigued. Accommodative response and dark focus are known to be influenced by stress (Westheimer 1957; Leibowitz, 1977), mood (Miller, 1978), refractive error (Maddock et al., 1981), and age (Bentivegna et al., 1981).

No data were reported on the normal individual variability in accommodative response or dark focus. The latency of the accommodative response and the rate at which it can be changed are known to vary between subjects and for the same subject under different conditions (see Chapter 7). It is thought that dark focus, which increased in this study by approximately 0.68 diopter following work, may exhibit a normal variability of 0.25 to 1 diopter in individual subjects over periods ranging from hours to days (Miller, 1978; Mershon and Amerson, 1980). Thus, the small changes in accommodative response or dark focus may not have been due solely to the visual stimulus.

The differences in the findings between the air traffic controllers and the other two groups are attributed in the report primarily to the more visually demanding work performed by the air traffic controllers. There are several problematic aspects to this interpretation. The data for the two telephone groups--each of which performed a different type of task, with a different amount of actual VDT work, presumably in a different working environment (the working environments were not described), on a different type of video display of unreported design--were pooled, and the average values were compared with average values obtained for the air traffic controllers, who performed tasks of a different nature for a specified period of time (2 hours), used video displays that are not typical of most VDTs, and worked in different environments than either of the two telephone groups. Because the three groups were not matched on any of these variables, the effects of differences in visual tasks are confounded with the effects of differences in many other variable s; thus, it is not possible to attribute the findings to the more visually demanding work of the air traffic controllers.

Even though the findings for the two telephone groups were reported as <u>not</u> statistically significant, Östberg concludes that "distance myopia" and "near hyperopia" occurred in these groups and appears to attribute this to the use of VDTs. Even if the findings had been statistically significant, it would not be possible to assess the relationship between the reported changes and use of VDTs because no control groups of non-VDT workers were included in this study.

Appendix B

Review of a Preliminary Report on a Cross-Sectional Survey of VDT Users at the *Baltimore Sun*

R. Van Harrison

This paper contains three major sections: the first section is the summary from the NIOSH study (Smith et al., 1982), the second summarizes and comments on the approach and methods of the study, and the third considers conclusions to be drawn from the study.

SUMMARY OF THE NIOSH STUDY

The National Institute of Occupational Safety and Health, was asked by a representative of employees of the Newspaper Guild, AFL-CIO, representing a large segment of employees at the Baltimore Sunpapers, to undertake an evaluation of the effects of video display terminals (VDTs) "on the environment and health of employees who use them."

Included in the request was the statement that there had occurred "several cases of cataracts among VDT users, a high rate of complaints about eye problems such as irritation and blurred vision and headaches, back and neck aches . . .(sic)" Accordingly, we undertook a cross-sectional survey, to define the type of eye and body complaints reported by VDT users, and to identify their relation to VDT use; the association between symptoms and the participants' abilities to see clearly (i.e., their refractive abilities relative to the demands for clear vision required by their job); and the prevalence of eye abnormalities, including cataracts and retinal abnormalities, and their relationship to VDT use.

R. Van Harrison, who is a study director at the Institute for Social Research at the University of Michigan, was a consultant to the panel.

We surveyed 379 employees of the Baltimore Sun, 283 of whom were members of the Newspaper Guild. Each participant answered a self-administered questionnaire on personal and job information, symptom complaints, and on a personal assessment of the pressure, pace, autonomy, and security, and satisfaction associated with the job. Each survey participant underwent a complete eye examination.

Using a statistical technique known as "factor analysis", we found that as participants increasingly reported that they were bothered by the brightness of the VDT screen or characters, by the glare off the screen, by the readability of the characters, or by flicker; they also increasingly reported (1) changes in their visual function, namely, seeing colored fringes around objects, difficulty reading and focusing on characters; (2) pain and stiffness in their neck, shoulders, and back; (3) headaches associated with work, in particular their usual job; and (4) headaches accompanied by itching, burning, watery eyes, blurry vision, nasal discharge and sweating. As participants tended to report that their VDT use typically involved shifting their eyes between the source document, VDT keyboard and screen; and as they tended to report that they found that they were bothered by the relative height, distance, and tilt of the VDT keyboard and screen; so too they tended to report that their headaches characteristically were superficial in location, dull and boring in sensation, beginning on one side of the head, but spreading to involve both sides. As participants reported a greater total number of years of VDT operating experience, they tended to report less that their headaches occurred during periods of stress, worry, and/or tension. As participants reported a greater number of hours per week of VDT operation, they also tended to report less that their headaches were preceded and accompanied by double and blurry vision. Controlling in the analyses for other characteristics of the participants, which might affect the symptoms being reported, did not change these observed associations in any meaningful way.

We did not find any meaningful relationship between adequacy of the participants' refractions, including the wearing of glasses with bi- or multifocal lenses, and the reporting of work-associated symptoms. We did not find any signficiant association between VDT use, including hours per week of VDT operation and total years of VDT operating experience; and the prevalence of eye abnormalities, including cataracts.

We note that among VDT users, the average number of years of VDT operating experience was 3.8 years, with a maximum of 9.2 years. If a minimum duration of VDT usage is postulated to be required prior to eye abnormalities being detectable, then the group of participants in this survey may well be judged to have had an insufficient amount of VDT usage for us to have found any such postulated associations. Therefore, our survey may well have been inadequate in terms of amount of exposure to resolve such issues as the putative associations of cataracts and VDT usage.

This survey has been primarily of value in delineating the relationship between VDT-users' symptoms and various ergonomic aspects of VDT use. The bothersome visual aspects of the VDT itself, as usually adjusted, explained the plurality of work-associated symptoms, even when other participant and work place characteristics were taken into account. We suggest that future emphasis be placed on research in regard to VDT viewing characteristics, and other aspects of the VDT viewing environment. We feel that these problems are best addressed experimentally.

REVIEW OF THE NIOSH STUDY

Study Approach and Methods

Introduction and Background

The study report begins with a review of related literature, identifying from previous studies important variables associated with VDT use and possible health problems. The organization of the analyses and discussion indicates an underlying conceptual model of categories of variables and their expected relationships; however, this model is not explicitly presented in the report.

Design

The study was performed to identify relationships between VDT use and health problems. It was an exploratory effort, attempting a more rigorous control of confounding factors than has been performed in previous studies. A cross-sectional field study was performed. A population of convenience was identified at the Baltimore Sun--convenient because of the high level of VDT use among the staff and some indication of health problems potentially related to VDT use. This population does not necessarily represent any other VDT user population, so findings must be generalized with caution. Indeed, the 49 percent participation rate of the eligible Newspaper Guild members and comparisons between demographic characteristics of participants and some nonparticipants suggest some differences between participants and nonparticipants. For example, the participants were more likely to use a VDT on the job and tended to have more formal education than the nonparticipants. The size of the main analysis sample, Newspaper Guild members who were VDT users ($N = 283$), and the various subsamples is adequate to detect with confidence somewhat weak relationships, for example, correlations of .25 in the main analysis sample.

The design, sample, and sample size are appropriate for exploring possible relationships between VDT use and health problems in a group likely to be at risk. The causal direction reflected in associations cannot be inferred from the data. The sample size is too small to test for increases in very infrequent health problems. These design limitations are clearly indicated in the report.

Measures

One of the important strengths of the study is the variety of variables included in it: aspects of VDT use; characteristics of the individuals, including demographic characteristics and use of bifocal or multifocal lenses; characteristics of the job, including the work setting (especially lighting) and job characteristics; and health problems, including headaches and other symptoms, and abnormal ophthalmologic findings. Of course, no one study can include all potentially relevant variables. For example, this study does not measure workers' skills in using VDTs.

Most data are obtained from self-report questionnaires. Clinically specific data, including visual characteristics, refraction, lenses, and other findings, are obtained from an ophthalmologic examination. The self-report data provide information concerning a wide range of variables for relatively little cost. The associated disadvantage is that the data are limited to users' perceptions and users' accuracy in reporting them. For example, people may differ in their reports concerning the flickering of a screen or an illumination contrast. Other studies must determine the extent to which differing reports reflect individual differences in perception and accommodation or other differences in aspects of the work. The measures are certainly adequate to indicate the most likely problems as perceived by the workers.

The two instruments, questionnaire and ophthalmologic exam form, appear to be fairly standard, drawn largely from previous instruments. Information on the source of the items would provide a perspective on specific results, particularly if some comparable data were available for specific items. The data collection procedures are fairly standard. The Saturday appointment for the exam may account for some of the nonparticipation rate.

The report does not present much data concerning the reliability of the measures. The factor analyses performed to produce several of the multiple item measures indicate the internal consistency of the measures. A more specific examination of the agreement among items within the final multiple item measures could have been obtained by calculating the coefficient (alpha) for each measure. No report of interexaminer agreement was presented.

Analyses

A consistent and well-thought-out analysis plan was followed to describe the range of findings, identify correlations (and therefore potential confounding) between variables, and carry out multivariate analyses of the effects of predictor variables on outcomes.

The distributions of scores are indicated for all measures except those variables derived through factor analysis and reported as standard scores. Although the standard scores are useful for relative comparisons, they provide little information concerning the range of scores on the original scales (typically a 6-point scale ranging from "never" to "always"). For example, the reported data provide no indication of the distribution of scores for time spent with "eyes fixed" on the screen or for frequency of various headache symptoms.

The analyses investigating relationships among variables are very well planned. Systematic checking for possible confounding, forward and backward replication of stepwise analyses, and attempts to cross-validate the results in a separate sample evidence a careful and critical examination of the data.

Conclusions

The authors of the study are careful to point out the major limitations of the study design and to counsel caution in drawing conclusions.

Substantive Conclusions

In this study, simply using a VDT was not automatically associated with health problems. However, particular aspects of VDT use were associated with types of headaches and other symptoms: poor visual clarity of the screen and improper lighting of the workplace were the most apparent. Their relationships to somatic symptoms were generally independent of the effects of other variables. The importance of VDT screen clarity is underscored by this association of VDT clarity with work-related headaches and with changes in visual functioning. These two relationships were the only findings replicated in a small, independent sample of non-guild VDT users. The authors appropriately recommend that future studies emphasize visual aspects of VDTs and workplace lighting, two factors that directly affect the viewing process.

Three other variables related to VDT use had significant independent relationships with one or another of the headache measures. Two of the variables reflect quantitative use of VDTs (years of experience, hours per week of VDT operations), and the third variable ("eyes shifting" mode of use) reflects a qualitative pattern associated with VDT use.

The relationships between the quantitative use of VDTs and headaches were negative, indicating more problems among less experienced users. This finding appears to contradict the simple hypothesis that VDT use automatically causes problems, with a greater amount of VDT use related to more problems. One explanation for the observed negative relationship would be that less skillful (i.e., less experienced) VDT operators are more likely to have problems operating VDTs, resulting in more problems for them. Future studies will need to examine variables likely to account for this negative relationship.

The relationship between the qualitative use of VDTs ("eyes shifting") and headaches was positive. This finding is difficult to interpret because eyes shifting was associated with work that was demanding with little time to do it (job attitude factor 1). Although this job factor was not related to the particular type of headache measure to which the eyes shifting mode was related, the job factor was related to three other headache and symptom measures. Future studies will have to determine the extent to which the underlying causal effects are due to the pattern of eye movements required with VDT use or the job characteristics of individuals who use the VDT in this mode.

An important "nonfinding" was that there was no significant difference between VDT workers and non-VDT workers on the items in the ophthalmologic examination. The authors point out the limitations of the study in that causal processes may take longer than the exposure of the study sample to VDTs and that the sample size is too small to detect infrequent (but important) negative outcomes. The more positive conclusion to be drawn from the study is that an average of 3.8 years of operating VDTs did not produce a sizable increase in negative ophthalmological findings. Studies to detect longer-term effects, very infrequent events, or smaller effects will have to be specially designed for those purposes.

Another set of nonfindings concerns wearing bifocal or multi-focal glasses: their use was not associated with any significant increase in headaches or symptoms. Wearing such glasses does not appear to have a sizable impact on headaches or other somatic symptoms.

An unfortunate omission in the presentation of results is an indication of the extent to which headaches and somatic symptoms are a problem among VDT users. It was noted in the previous section that means on these measures (along with all of the measures developed through factor analysis) are reported only as standard scores. While the original scale is somewhat difficult to interpret (a 6-point scale ranging from "never" to "always"), transforming the mean standard scores to this scale would present some information concerning the magnitude of the effect involved. For example, the positive relationship between workstation lighting and pain and stiffness in the axial muscula-ture would be more important to pursue if the pain and stiffness scores for individuals with poor lighting averaged 5 rather than 1.5 on the original 6-point scale. All of the significant relationships with outcomes are with the symptom variables. Although the report identifies the variables associated with these outcomes, it does not indicate the frequency or severity of these outcomes in the study sample.

Methodological Conclusions and Limitations

The study findings confirm methodological refinements that must be incorporated into subsequent studies of VDT use. Separate and distinct measures of the frequency of operating in an "eyes fixed" mode and an "eyes shifting" mode must be made. Similarly, dis-tinct measures must be made between positional problems and visual problems associated with VDT use. These modes and problems have different relationships to demographic factors, job characteristics, and symptoms. The conceptual elaboration and refinement of activities associated with VDTs is shown to be a necessary activity in studies of VDTs. Additional distinctions concerning the types of work and types of user problems are likely to be productive.

The results indicated that confounding frequently occurred between VDT use measures, demographic factors, and job characteristics and attitudes. However, the effects of the variables were separable. The findings indicate that future studies should include presently identified confounding factors. For example, confounded demographic factors in relationships between measures of VDT use and measures of headache and somatic symptoms include educational level, years of employment, and age. Future studies should attempt to identify and control the effects of other potential confounding factors, such as a user's skills in using VDTs.

A methodological limitation of the findings is that the only significant relationships between VDT use and outcomes were found between self-reports of VDT use and self-reports concerning various symptoms. All survey studies may be affected by respondent perceptions and biases that introduce or alter relationships. However, in the present study, the findings generally follow expected patterns, evidence differential relationships, and are generally interpretable, indicating the construct validity of the measures.

The limitations on the generalizability of the preceding conclusions were noted in the discussion of the study sample. The conclusions cannot automatically be generalized to any other population. However, in the absence of other information, factors that are more important in this population should certainly have a priority for further study in other populations. The relationship between VDT use and health outcomes is complex because of the range of possibilities in VDT work, relevant health outcomes, and confounding personal and job factors.

As in any applied area, future research must include a number of methodological approaches. Broad, exploratory studies similar to the present study must be performed in other populations to determine the replicability of relationships and problem magnitude across individuals, jobs, and VDT equipment. More expensive methodologies (e.g., direct observations of VDT use, health diaries) should be used to collect more detailed data on variables of interest. Longitudinal studies can help clarify causal relationships. Experimental studies will both clarify causal relationships and evaluate possible improvements in VDT use. The authors of the report specifically recommend that effects of workplace lighting and of visual clarity of the screen now be systematically investigated in experimental studies. The convergence of findings from cross-sectional survey studies will help identify the most important variables to study and to control in laboratory and field experiments to reduce problems associated with VDT use.

Dissent

Lawrence W. Stark

I am dissenting from our panel report because of my concern that the report does not provide adequate guidance to a VDT user or his or her physician regarding complaints of ocular discomfort and visual fatigue. I do not, however, disagree with the body of the report or with the "Executive Summary" in any of the detailed findings; in particular, I do not believe that radiation damage or serious diseases such as cataracts result from VDT use.

My own review of the literature substantiated the opinion that visual fatigue is not a well-defined physiological or clinical entity, but this scientifically accurate statement cannot negate the fact that all of us feel fatigue at various times. Indeed, many of us, finding ourselves at a given moment without sufficient motivation to go on, have halted tasks as a result of fatigue. I believe that many highly motivated VDT users suffer from ocular discomfort and visual fatigue beyond that appropriate to a normal workplace.

Implicit in the appearance of video display terminals on the marketplace for office and clerical work is the manufacturers' claim that adequate legibility can be obtained from these terminals. I believe this not to be true. I have never seen a video display terminal that was nearly as legible as the ordinary pieces of typewritten paper or copied reports that circulate in our paper world. We all prefer to look down, with easy convergence on reading matter--a book, a sheet of typewritten material, or handwritten correspondence. No VDTs provide robust enough contrast to enable this "natural" position for the tube face. Most commercially available VDTs have been simply adapted from television entertainment video monitors. Those monitors were originally designed for pictures with fairly large images and especially for images in motion, a quite different spatial resolution task than reading static alphanumeric characters. Also, consideration must be given to the length of time spent at a task and the possible inflexibility of a job requiring reading from the face of a VDT for an 8-hour day. Our panel report does not condemn the poor quality and legibility of current VDTs, but rather states that scientific evaluation is difficult.

These deficiencies in the report may be the result of the process by which the report was assembled. The charges to the panel (listed in the preface) are narrowly directed. The panel, excellent scientists from the academic community, all thoroughly reviewed the scientific literature. We met face to face as a panel on four occasions and also had opportunities to attend several related professional meetings in Washington, D.C. Thus, adequate time and effort was spent sharing each others' partitioned reviews forming the narrow responses to the charges; I learned about ergonomics, display technology, job design, survey methodology, radiation standards, and clinical epidemiology. In contrast, adequate time was not spent on consideration of policy questions by the group as a whole (time and funding constraints, not conspiracy, determined this). As I learned more about these issues and realized how central they were to the panel's overall tasks, I missed the luxury of panel face-to-face discussions on them. Rather a complex procedure, all by correspondence, of multiple review and responsive modifications ensued. Thus the panel, to my frustration, was unable to deal as a group with interpretation and policy, but remained limited to our focused scientific reviews in response to the narrow charges. My dissent rests on possible misinterpretation of the report with its detailed, balanced "scientific" outlook and style, as supporting the status quo of no standards or guidelines for VDT workplaces and no clear concern with unacceptable levels of ocular discomfort and visual fatigue.

Biographical Sketches of Panel Members and Staff

EDWARD J. RINALDUCCI is professor of psychology and coordinator of the Engineering Psychology Program at the school of psychology of the Georgia Institute of Technology. Previously he held academic positions at the University of Virginia. His current research interests include both basic and applied aspects of vision research, illuminating engineering, human factors in transportation systems (i.e., automobile and aircraft), and human spatial behavior. He is a member of the American Psychological Association, the Human Factors Society, the Optical Society of America, the Illuminating Engineering Society, the Association of Aviation Psychologists, the Psychonomic Society, and Sigma Xi. He received a BA degree in psychology from Lehigh University, an MA degree from the University of New Hampshire, and a PhD degree in psychology from the University of Rochester.

JANET BERTINUSON is director of occupational health and safety for the Alberta Federation of Labour, and she serves on the Canadian Labour Congress National Health and Safety Committee and the Labour Canada Committee on the labeling of hazardous substances. Previously she was acting director of the Labor Occupational Health Program at the University of California, Berkeley, and health and safety associate for the Oil, Chemical and Atomic Workers International Union. She has a BA degree from Clarke College and an MS degree in environmental health from the University of Cincinnati.

ROBERT D. CAPLAN is senior study director at the Institute for Social Research at the University of Michigan. His research interests and publications deal with psychosocial stressors, particularly in work settings, and how these stressors affect mental and physical health. He is a fellow of the Section on

237

Epidemiology of the American Heart Association, a past officer of
the Society for the Social Psychological Study of Social Issues
(Division 9 of the American Psychological Association), and a
former Fulbright scholar. He received a PhD degree in
organizational psychology from the University of Michigan.

ROBERT M. GUION is university professor of psychology at
Bowling Green State University. He has been at Bowling Green
since receiving his PhD in 1952, except for periods of leave to
teach at the University of California, Berkeley, and the University of New Mexico and to do research for the state of Hawaii and
the Educational Testing Service. His research interests are primarily in the field of industrial and organizational psychology,
more specifically in the study of fair employment practices in
employee selection and employee compensation. He has served as
chair of the Board of Scientific Affairs of the American Psychological Association (APA) and has been the president of two
divisions in the APA. He is editor of the Journal of Applied
Psychology. He has twice received the James McKeen Cattell
award for excellence in research design. He did his undergraduate
work at the State University of Iowa and received a PhD degree
from Purdue University.

VINCENT M. KING is associate dean of the College of Optometry
at Ferris State College. Previously he held faculty positions at
Ohio State University and Pennsylvania College of Optometry. He
has also served as chairman of the Commission on Ophthalmic
Standards of the American Optometric Association and as the
organization's representative on various American National
Standards Institute committees charged with developing ophthalmic standards. His research interests include study of the physiological bases of ocular and visually related discomfort. He is a
fellow of the American Academy of Optometry and a member of
the American Optometric Association and the Association for
Research in Vision and Ophthalmology. He received a BSc degree
in optometry and MSc and PhD degrees from Ohio State University.

DAVID H. SLINEY is chief of the Laser Branch, Laser Microwave
Division, of the U.S. Army Environmental Hygiene Agency at
Aberdeen Proving Ground, Maryland. He has published widely on
subjects related to laser hazards and is an editor of Health
Physics. He is a subcommittee chairman on the American
National Standards Institute (ANSI) committees on safe use of

lasers and on safety of lights and lighting systems and is chairman of the safety committee of the Laser Institute of America. He was a U.S. delegate to the committee on lasers of the International Electrotechnical Commission and was also a participant in a meeting on lasers of the World Health Organization. He is a member of the Optical Society of America, the American Society of Photobiology, the Health Physics Society, the Society of Photo-Optical Instrumentation Engineers, the American Industrial Hygiene Association, the Association for Research in Vision and Ophthalmology, and the physical agent committee of the American Conference of Governmental Industrial Hygienists. He received a BS degree in physics from Virginia Polytechnic Institute and an MS degree in physics from Emory University.

STANLEY W. SMITH is professor emeritus at Ohio State University. He participates in the university's sensory biophysics program and is a member of the zoology department and the Institute for Research in Vision. Previously he held research positions at the Engineering Psychology Laboratory and the Vision Research Laboratories of the Universty of Michigan. For the past 12 years most of his research has involved relationships between lighting variables, age, subjective ratings, and performance of common visual tasks such as reading and verifying columns of numbers. He serves on two technical committees, on visual performance and on visual environment, of the Commission Internationale de l'Eclairage. He received BA and MA degrees from Oberlin College and a PhD from the University of Michigan, all in psychology.

HARRY L. SNYDER is professor of industrial engineering and operations research at Virginia Polytechnic Institute and State University, where he established the human factors graduate program in 1970. Previously he held research positions at North American Rockwell Corporation and the Boeing Company. His research has focused on visual display evaluation and visual problems of an applied nature, and he has published extensively in the general human factors engineering field, with particular emphasis on visual performance. In 1981 he received the Paul M. Fitts Award from the Human Factors Society for his contributions to human factors education. He is a fellow of the Human Factors Society, the Optical Society of America, and the American Psychological Association. He has served as president and as a member of the executive council of the Human Factors Society and editor of Human Factors. He received an AB degree from Brown University and MA and PhD degrees from Johns Hopkins University.

ALFRED SOMMER is associate professor of ophthalmology, epidemiology, and international health at Johns Hopkins University and director of the International Center for Epidemiologic and Preventive Ophthalmology, a World Health Organization Collaborating Center for the Prevention of Blindness, in Baltimore. He also serves as medical advisor of Helen Keller International. His major research interests concern epidemiologic and public health analyses of ocular and blinding disorders. He has received the Helen Keller International Blindness Prevention Award. He is chairman of the Public Health Committee of the American Academy of Ophthalmology, has served on consultative and advisory bodies of the National Institutes of Health, the Institute on Nutrition and Aging, and the World Health Organization, and is a member of the American Academy of Ophthalmology, the Royal Society of Medicine, the Society for Epidemiologic Research, the Association for Research in Vision and Ophthalmology, the American College of Preventive Medicine, and the American Public Health Association. He received a BS degree from Union College, an MD degree from Harvard Medical School, and an MHSc degree in epidemiology from the Johns Hopkins School of Hygiene and Public Health.

LAWRENCE W. STARK is a professor of physiological optics and engineering science at the University of California, Berkeley, and professor of neurology (neuroophthalmology) at the University of California Medical Center, San Francisco. Previously he was at Yale University School of Medicine and the Massachusetts Institute of Technology. His interest in neurological control systems has focused on eye movements and their role in vision. He is the author of Neurological Control Systems (1968) and more than 200 scientific articles. He received an AB degree from Columbia College and an MD degree from Albany Medical College.

H. LEE TASK is a research physicist in the field of optics at the Human Engineering Division of the Air Force Aerospace Medical Research Laboratory. His research interests and work include display image quality measurement and assessment, helmet mounted displays, night vision imaging devices and aids, aircraft windscreen optical quality measurement, and human visual performance. He has authored many papers and articles and holds several patents in these and related areas. He is a member of the Optical Society of America and the Human Factors Society. He received a BS degree in physics from Ohio University, an MS degree in physics from Purdue University, and MS and PhD

degrees in optical sciences from the University of Arizona Optical
Sciences Center.

HUGH R. TAYLOR is assistant professor of ophthalmology, epidemiology, and international health at Johns Hopkins University
and assistant director of the International Center for Epidemiologic and Preventive Ophthalmology, a World Health Organization
Collaborating Center for the Prevention of Blindness, in Baltimore. His major research interests concern the epidemiologic and
public health analyses of ocular and blinding disorders and the
immunopathogenesis of blinding ocular infections. He is currently
a member of an expert advisory panel and a scientific working
group of the World Health Organization, and he has served on
consultative and advisory bodies of the National Institutes of
Health; the International Vitamin A Consultative Group sponsored
by the U.S. Agency for International Development; the National
Health and Medical Research Council, Australia; and the World
Health Organization. He has received the citation for clinical
research given by Fight For Sight, Inc., and the Association for
Research in Vision and Ophthalmology. He is a member of the
American Academy of Ophthalmology, the American Medical
Association, the American Society of Tropical Medicine and
Hygiene, the Association for Research in Vision and Ophthal-
mology, the Royal Australian College of Surgeons, the Royal
Australian College of Ophthalmologists, and the Royal Society of
Medicine. He received an MS-BS degree, a BMedSci degree, a DO
degree, and an MD degree in ophthalmic epidemiology from the
University of Melbourne.

KEY DISMUKES is study director of the Committee on Vision and
served as study director to the panel. His publications cover a
range of topics in neuroscience and in science and public policy.
He is a member of the International Brain Research Organization
and the Society for Neuroscience, in which he has served on or
chaired several committees. He received a BS degree from North
Georgia College, an MA degree from Vanderbilt University, and a
PhD degree in biophysics from Pennsylvania State University.

BARBARA S. BROWN served as staff associate to the panel and is
now research associate in the Institute of Medicine. Previously
she held positions in several divisions of the National Research
Council. She has a BA degree in psychology and zoology from
George Washington University.

References

Able, L., Dell'Oso, L. F., Daroff, R. A., and Parker, L.
1979   Saccades in extremes of gaze. Investigative Ophthalmology
         18:324-327.
Acton, W. I., and Carson, M. B.
1967   Auditory and subjective effects of airborne noise from
         industrial ultrasonic sources. British Journal of Industrial
         Medicine 24:297-305.
Adler-Grinberg, D., and Stark, L.
1978   Eye movements, scanpaths, and dyslexia. American Journal
         of Optometry and Physiological Optics 55:557-570.
Allen, M. J.
1955   The stimulus to accommodation. American Journal of
         Optometry 32:422-431.
American Conference of Governmental Industrial Hygienists
1981   Threshold Limit Values for Chemical Substances and
         Physical Agents in the Workroom Environment with Intended
         Changes for 1981. Cincinnati: American Conference of
         Governmental Industrial Hygienists.
Andersson, G. J., and Ortengren, R.
1974   Lumbar disc pressure and myoelectric back muscle activity
         during sitting. Scandinavian Journal of Rehabilitation
         3:115-121.
1979   Belastningen pa ryggen vid olika utformning av stolar. Pp.
         33-59 in B. Johsson, G. Andersson, G. Hedberg, J. Winkel,
         and S. Engdahl, eds., Sittande Arbetsstallningar. Report No.
         1978:12. Umea, Sweden: Arbetarskyddsstyrelsen.
Applied Ergonomics
1970   Seating in industry. Applied ergonomics handbook. Part 1.
         Applied Ergonomics 1(3):159-165.
Arndt, R.
1981   Telephone Operator Reactions to Video Display Terminals.
         Paper presented at American Industrial Hygiene Association
         conference, Portland, Oregon, May.
Association for Computing Machinery, Washington, D.C., Chapter, and
the Institute for Computer Sciences and Technology of the National
Bureau of Standards
1982   Proceedings: Human Factors in Computer Systems. March
         15-17, Gaithersburg, Md. Washington, D.C.: Association for
         Computing Machinery, Washington, D.C., Chapter.

243

Astrand, P. O., and Rodahl, K.
    1977   Textbook of Work Physiology. New York: McGraw-Hill.
Ayoub, M. M., and Halcomb, C. G.
    1976   Improved Seat, Console, and Workplace Design. Pacific
            Missile Test Center, Report No. TP-76-1. Point Mugu,
            Calif.: Department of the Navy.
Bach-y-Rita, P.
    1971   Neurophysiology of eye movements. Pp. 7-45 in P.
            Bach-y-Rita, C. C. Collins, and J. E. Hyde, eds., The Control
            of Eye Movements. New York: Academic Press.
Bagnara, M.
    1980   Error detection at visual display units. Pp. 142-146 in E.
            Grandjean and E. Vigliani, eds., Ergonomic Aspects of Visual
            Display Terminals. London: Taylor & Francis.
Bahill, A. T., and Stark, L.
    1975   Overlapping saccades and glissades are produced by fatigue
            in the saccadic eye movement system. Experimental
            Neurology 48:95-106.
Bahill, A. T., Ciuffreda, K. J., Kenyon, R., and Stark, L.
    1976   Dynamic and static violations of Hering's law of equal
            innervation. American Journal of Optometry and
            Physiological Optics 53:786-796.
Bales, R. F.
    1950   Interaction Process Analysis. Cambridge, Mass.:
            Addison-Wesley.
Baloh, R. W., and Honrubia, V.
    1979   Clinical Neurophysiology of the Vestibular System. Vol. 18.
            Philadelphia: F. A. Davis.
Barlow, H. B., and Andrews, D. P.
    1973   The site at which rhodopsin bleaching raises the scotopic
            threshold. Vision Research 13:903-908.
Barmack, N. H., and Pettorosi, V. E.
    1980   Vestibulo ocular reflex in rabbits—reduction by intravenous
            injection of diazepam. Archives of Neurology 37:718-722.
Barnowe, J. T., Mangione, T. W., and Quinn, R. P.
    1973   Quality of employment indicators, occupational
            classifications, and demographic characteristics as
            predictors of job satisfaction. Pp. 385-392 in R. P. Quinn
            and T. W. Mangione, eds., The 1969-1970 Survey of Working
            Conditions: Chronicles of an Unfinished Enterprise. Ann
            Arbor: Institute for Social Research, University of
            Michigan.
Bartley, S. H.
    1938   Subjective brightness in relation to flash rate and the
            light-dark ratio. Journal of Experimental Psychology
            23:313-319.
    1942   A factor in visual fatigue. Psychosomatic Medicine
            4:369-375.
Bauer, D., and Cavonius, C. R.
    1980   Improving the legibility of visual display units through
            contrast reversal. Pp. 137-142 in E. Grandjean and E.
            Vigliani, eds., Ergonomic Aspects of Visual Display
            Terminals. London: Taylor & Francis.

Beamon, W. S., and Snyder, H. L.
  1980   An Experimental Evaluation of the Spot Wobble Method of
          Suppressing Raster Structure Visibility. Aerospace Medical
          Laboratory Technical Report No. AMRL-75-63. Dayton,
          Ohio: Wright-Patterson Air Force Base.
Bear, J. D., and Richler, A.
  1982   Environmental influences on ocular refraction. American
          Journal of Epidemiology 115:138-139.
Bedell, R. J.
  1975   Modulation transfer function of very high resolution
          miniature cathode ray tubes. Proceedings of the Society for
          Information Display 16(3):212-215.
Bender, M. B., and Shanzer, S.
  1964   Oculomotor pathways defined by electric stimulation and
          lesions in the brain stem of monkeys. Pp. 81-140 in M. B.
          Bender, ed., The Oculomotor System. New York: Harper &
          Row.
Bentivegna, J., Owens, D. A., and Messner, K.
  1981   Aging, cycloplegia, and the accuracy of accommodation.
          Investigative Ophthalmology and Visual Science 20(3):21.
Berens, C., and Sells, S.
  1954   Experimental studies on fatigue of accommodation. I.
          Archives of Ophthalmology 31:148-159.
Berens, C., and Stark, E. K.
  1932   Studies in ocular fatigue. IV. Fatigue of accommodation,
          experimental and clinical observations. American Journal of
          Ophthalmology 15:527-542.
Bergman, T.
  1980   Health effects of video display terminals. Occupational
          Health and Safety. November/December: 25-28, 53-55.
Berlyne, D. E.
  1958   The influence of complexity and novelty in visual figures on
          orienting responses. Journal of Experimental Psychology
          55:286-289.
Bitterman, M. E.
  1945   Heart rate and frequency of blinking as indices of visual
          efficiency. Journal of Experimental Psychology 35:279-292.
  1946   A reply to Dr. Luckiesh. Journal of Experimental
          Psychology 36:182-184.
  1947   Frequency of blinking in visual work: a reply to Dr.
          Luckiesh. Journal of Experimental Psychology 37:269-270.
Blatt, N.
  1931   Weakness of accommodation. Archives of Ophthalmology
          62:372-373.
Boghen, D., Troost, B. T., Daroff, R. A., Dell'Oso, L. F., and Birkett, J. E.
  1974   Velocity characteristics of normal human saccades.
          Investigative Ophthalmology 13:619-622.
Booker, R. L.
  1981   Luminance-brightness comparisons of separated circular
          stimuli. Journal of the Optical Society of America
          71:139-144.
Borish, I. M.
  1970   Clinical Refraction. Vol. 1. Chicago: Professional Press.

Bouma, H.
  1980   Visual reading processes and the quality of text displays. Pp.
          101-114 in E. Grandjean and E. Vigliani, eds., Ergonomic
          Aspects of Visual Display Terminals. London: Taylor &
          Francis.
Bourough, H. C., Warnock, R. F., and Britt, J. H.
  1967   Quantitative Determination of Image Quality. Report No.
          2-114058-1. Seattle: Boeing Aircraft Co.
Bowers, D. G., and Hauser, D. L.
  1977   Work group types and intervention effects in organizational
          development. Administrative Science Quarterly 22:76-94.
Bowers, D. G., and Seashore, S. E.
  1966   Predicting organizational effectiveness with a four-factor
          theory of leadership. Administrative Science Quarterly
          11:238-263.
Boynton, R. M.
  1961   Some temporal factors in vision. Pp. 739-756 in W. A.
          Rosenblith, ed., Sensory Communications. New York: John
          Wiley & Sons.
Boynton, R. M., and Miller, N. D.
  1963   Visual performance under conditions of transient adap-
          tation. Illuminating Engineering 58:541-550.
Boynton, R. M., Rinalducci, E. J., and Sternheim, C. E.
  1969   Visibility losses produced by transient adaptational changes
          in the range from 0.4 to 4000 Foot-Lamberts. Illuminating
          Engineering 64:217-227.
Branton, P., and Grayson, G.
  1967   An evaluation of train seats by observation of sitting
          behavior. Ergonomics 12:316-327.
Brehm, J. W.
  1966   A Theory of Psychological Reactance. New York:
          Academic Press.
Breland, K., and Breland, M. K.
  1944   Legibility of newspaper headlines printed in capitals and in
          lower case. Journal of Applied Psychology 28:117-120.
Brown, B. S., Dismukes, R. K., and Rinalducci, E. J.
  1982   Video display terminals and vision of workers. Summary and
          overview of a symposium. Behaviour and Information
          Technology 1(2):121-140.
Brown, C. R., and Schaum, D. L.
  1980   User-adjusted VDU parameters. Pp. 195-200 in E. Grandjean
          and E. Vigliani, eds., Ergonomic Aspects of Visual Display
          Terminals. London: Taylor & Francis.
Brozek, J., Simonson, E., and Keys, A.
  1950   Changes in performance and in ocular functions resulting
          from strenuous visual inspection. American Journal of
          Psychology 63:51-66.
Bureau of Radiological Health
  1981   An Evaluation of Radiation Emission from Video Display
          Terminals. HHS Publication No. FDA 81-8153. Washington,
          D.C.: Department of Health and Human Services.
Burger, J. M., and Cooper, H. M.
  1979   The desirability of control. Motivation and Emotion
          3:381-393.

Caird, F. I.
1973   Problems of cataract epidemiology with special reference to
        diabetes. Pp. 281-301 in A. Pirie, ed., Symposium on the
        Human Lens in Relation to Cataract, London, 1973. Ciba
        Foundation Symposium No. 19. Amsterdam: Elsevier.
Cakir, A., Reuter, H.-J., von Schmude, L., and Armbruster, A.
1978   Untersuchungen zur Anpassung von Bildschirmarbeitsplatzen
        an die Physische und Psychische Funktionsweise des
        Menschen. Bonn, Germany: Der Bundersminister für Arbeit
        und Sozialordnung.
Cakir, A., Hart, D. J., and Stewart, T. F. M.
1980   Visual Display Terminals. A Manual Covering Ergonomics,
        Workplace Design, Health and Safety, Task Organization.
        New York: John Wiley & Sons.
Cameron, C.
1973   A theory of fatigue. Ergonomics 16:633-648.
Campbell, F. W., and Gubisch, R. W.
1966   Optical quality of the human eye. Journal of Physiology
        186:558-578.
Campbell, F. W., and Robson, J. G.
1968   Application of Fourier analysis to the visibility of gratings.
        Journal of Physiology 197:551-556.
Canadian Labour Congress
1982   Toward a More Humanized Technology: Exploring the
        Impact of VDTs on the Health and Working Conditions of
        Canadian Office Workers. Ottawa: CLC Labour Education
        and Studies Center.
Caplan, R. D.
1971   Organizational Stress and Individual Strain: A Socio-
        Psychological Study of Risk Factors in Coronary Heart
        Disease Among Administrators, Engineers, and Scientists.
        PhD dissertation. Department of Psychology, University of
        Michigan. University Microfilms No. 72-14822.
1979   Social support, person-environment fit, and coping. Pp.
        89-137 in L. Ferman and J. Gordus, eds., Mental Health and
        the Economy. Kalamazoo, Mich: W. E. Upjohn Institute for
        Employment Research.
1983   Person-environment fit: past, present and future. Pp. 35-78
        in C. Cooper, ed., Stress Research: Where Do We Go From
        Here? London: John Wiley & Sons.
Caplan, R. D., and Jones, K. W.
1975   Effects of work load, role ambiguity, Type A personality on
        anxiety, depression, and heart rate. Journal of Applied
        Psychology 60:713-719.
Caplan, R. D., Cobb, S., French, J. R. P., Jr., Harrison, R. V., and
Pinneau, S. R., Jr.
1975   Job Demands and Worker Health. NIOSH Research Report,
        HEW Publication 75-160. Washington, D.C.: U.S.
        Department of Health, Education, and Welfare.
Caplan, R. D., Cobb, S., and French, J. R. P., Jr.
1979   White collar work load and cortisol: disruption of a
        circadian rhythm by job stress? Journal of Psychosomatic
        Research 23:181-192.

Caplan, R. D., Cobb, S., French, J. R. P., Jr., Harrison, R. V., and
Pinneau, S. R., Jr.
    1980   Job Demands and Worker Health: Main Effects and
             Occupational Differences. Ann Arbor: Institute for Social
             Research, University of Michigan.

Carlson, C. R., and Cohen, R. W.
    1978   A model for predicting the just-noticeable difference in
             image structure as a function of display modulation
             transfer. Society for Information Display 78 Digest
             (April):30-31.

Carmichael, L.
    1951-   Reading and visual work: a contribution to the technique
    1952   of experimentation on human fatigue. Proceedings of the
             New York Academy of Sciences 14:94-97.

Carmichael, L., and Dearborn, W. F.
    1947   Reading and Visual Fatigue. New York: Houghton Mifflin.

Carpenter, R. H. S.
    1977   Movements of the Eyes. London: Pion.

Center for Disease Control
    1980   Working with video display terminals: a preliminary
             health-risk evaluation. Morbidity and Mortality Weekly
             Report 29(25):307-308.

Centers for Disease Control
    1981   Cluster of spontaneous abortions, Dallas, Texas.
             Unpublished memorandum from the Family Planning
             Evaluation Division, Center for Health Promotion and
             Education, Centers for Disease Control, to the Director,
             Centers for Disease Control, May 11.

Chandler, J. S.
    1973   Viewing Device with Filter Means for Optimizing Image
             Quality. U.S. Patent No. 3,744,893.

Chatterjee, A., Milton, R. C., and Thyle, S.
    1982   Prevalence and etiology of cataract in Punjab. British
             Journal of Ophthalmology 66:35-42.

Christensen, M.
    1981   Lighting prescription for areas containing cathode ray tube
             (CRT) displays. Lighting Design and Application 11(5):23-25.

Churchill, E., Laubach, L. L., McConville, J. T., and Tebbetts., I.
    1978   Anthropometric Source Book. Vols. 1-3. National
             Aeronautics and Space Administration RP 1024. Yellow
             Springs, Ohio: Webb Associates; and Houston: National
             Aeronautics and Space Administration.

Cobb, P. W., and Moss, R. K.
    1925   Eye fatigue and its relation to light and work. Journal of the
             Franklin Institute 200:239-247.

Cobb, S.
    1976   Social support as a moderator of life stress. Psychosomatic
             Medicine 3:300-314.

Cobb, S., and Kasl, S. V.
    1977   Termination: The Consequences of Job Loss. DHEW
             Publication No. (NIOSH) 77-224. Washington, D.C.: U. S.
             Department of Health, Education, and Welfare.

Cobb, S., and Rose, R. M.
1973   Hypertension, peptic ulcer, and diabetes in air traffic
        controllers. Journal of the American Medical Association
        224:489-492.
Coe, J. B., Cuttle, K., McClellan, W. C., and Warden, N. J.
1980   Visual Display Units. A Review of the Potential Health
        Problems Associated with Their Use. Wellington, N.Z.:
        Regional Occupational Health Unit, New Zealand
        Department of Health.
Cohen, S.
1980   Aftereffects of stress on human performance and social
        behavior: a review of research and theory. Psychological
        Bulletin 88:82-108.
Cole, B. L.
1981   VDU's--not a new disease: a new challenge. Australian
        Journal of Optometry 64:24-27.
Collins, C. C.
1975   The human oculomotor system. Pp. 145-180 in G.
        Lennerstrand and P. Bach-y-Rita, eds., Brain Mechanisms of
        Ocular Motility. Oxford, England: Pergamon Press.
Commission Internationale de l'Eclairage
1975   Guide on Interior Lighting. CIE Publication No. 29. Paris:
        Bureau Central de la CIE.
1980   Proceedings of the Commission Internationale de l'Eclairage
        (CIE) 19th Session, Kyoto, Japan. CIE Publication No. 50.
        Paris: Bureau Central de la CIE.
1981   An Analytic Model for Describing the Influence of Lighting
        Parameters Upon Visual Performance. Vol. I: Technical
        Foundations. Vol. II: Summary and Application Guidelines.
        CIE Publication Nos. 19/2.1 and 19/2.2 (TC-3.1). Paris:
        Bureau Central de la CIE.
Cook, T. D., and Campbell, D. T.
1976   The design and conduct of quasi-experiments and true
        experiments in field settings. Pp. 223-326 in M. D.
        Dunnette, ed., Handbook of Industrial and Organizational
        Psychology. Chicago: Rand McNally.
Costanza, E. B.
1981   An Evaluation of a Method to Determine Suprathreshold
        Color Contrast on CRT Displays. MS thesis. Department of
        Industrial Engineering and Operations Research, Virginia
        Polytechnic Institute and State University.
Cox, E. A.
1980   Radiation emissions from visual display units. Pp. 25-38 in
        Health Hazards of VDUs? Papers Presented at a One-Day
        Conference Sponsored by the HUSAT Research Group,
        Loughborough, England, December 11, 1980. Loughborough,
        England: Loughborough University of Technology.
Czerski, P., Ostrowski, K., Shore, M. L., Silverman, C., Suess, M. J., and
Waldeskog, B., eds.
1974   Biological Effects and Health Hazards of Microwave
        Radiation. Proceedings of an International Symposium,
        Warsaw, 15-18 October, 1973. Warsaw: Polish Medical
        Publishers.

Dainoff, M. J.
1980   Visual fatigue in VDT operators. Pp. 95-99 in E. Grandjean
        and E. Vigliani, eds., Ergonomic Aspects of Visual Display
        Terminals. London: Taylor & Francis.
1982   Occupational stress factors in visual display terminal (VDT)
        operation: a review of empirical research. Behaviour and
        Information Technology 1(2):141-176.
Dainoff, M. J., Happ, A., and Crane, P.
1981   Visual fatigue and occupational stress in VDT operators.
        Human Factors 23(4):421-438.
Dainty, J. C. and Shaw, R.
1974   Image Science. New York: Academic Press.
Daniels, G. S.
1952   The "Average Man?" Technical Note WCRD 53-7. Dayton,
        Ohio: Wright Air Development Center, Wright-Patterson Air
        Force Base.
DeBoer, J. B.
1977   Performance and comfort in the presence of veiling
        reflections. Lighting Research and Technology 9(4):169-176.
de Lange, H.
1958   Research into the dynamic nature of the human fovea-cortex
        systems with intermittent and modulated light: I.
        Attenuation characteristics with white and colored light.
        Journal of the Optical Society of America 48:777-784.
DeMatteo, B., FitzRandolph, K., and Daynes, S.
1981   The Hazards of VDTs. Ontario: Ontario Public Service
        Employees Union.
Demilia, L.
1968   Visual fatigue and reading. Journal of Education 151:4-34.
DePalma, J. J., and Lowrey, E. M.
1962   Sine-wave and square-wave contrast sensitivity. Journal of
        the Optical Society of America 52:328-335.
Deutsches Institut für Normungen
1982   Kennwerte füer die Anpassung von Bildschirmarbeits-
        platzen au den Menschen. DIN Standard 66234. Berlin:
        BEUTH Verlag GmbH. (Values taken from these DIN
        standards have been widely circulated and used in 1982. It is
        not known if they have been formally adopted.)
Doll, R., and Jones, F. A.
1951   Occupational Factors in Aetiology of Gastric and Duodenal
        Ulcers. Medical Research Council Special Report Series.
        London: Her Majesty's Stationery Office.
Duke-Elder, S.
1969   Diseases of the lens and vitreous: glaucoma and hypotony.
        Pp. 148-157 in System of Ophthalmology, Vol. XI. London:
        H. Kimpton.
Duke-Elder, S., and Abrams, D.
1970   Ophthalmic Optics and Refraction. Vol. V in S. Duke-Elder,
        ed., System of Ophthalmology. St. Louis: C. V. Mosby.
Easterby, R., Kroemer, K. H. E., and Chaffin, D. B., eds.
1982   Anthropometry and Biomechanics: Theory and Applications.
        Proceedings of the NATO Symposium, Cambridge, England,
        July 1980. New York: Plenum Press.

Ederer, F., Hiller, R., and Taylor, H. R.
1981a   Senile lens changes and diabetes in two population studies.
        American Journal of Ophthalmology 91:381.
1981b   Reply to Sommer (letter). American Journal of Ophthal-
        mology 92:135.
Eisen, D. J.
1981   Supplementary Analysis and Observations on the University
        of Wisconsin Report on Health Conditions of VDT Operators
        at the New York Times. Unpublished report prepared for the
        Newspaper Guild.
Electronics Industries Association
1957   Electrical Performance Standards--Monochrome Television
        Studio Facility. RS-170. Washington, D.C.: Electronics
        Industries Association.
Elias, R., Cail, F., Tisserand, M., and Christmann, H.
1980   Investigations in operators working with CRT display
        terminals: relationships between task content and
        psychophysiological alterations. Pp. 211-217 in E. Grandjean
        and E. Vigliani, eds., Ergonomic Aspects of Visual Display
        Terminals. London: Taylor & Francis.
Elias, R., Mayer, A., Cail, F., Christmann, H., and Barlier, A.
1979   Conditions de Travail Devant les Ecrans Cathodiques.
        Problemes lies a la Charge Visuelle. Report No. 1216-97-79.
        Paris: Institut National de Recherche et de Securite.
Emery, F. E., and Trist, E. L.
1960   Management Science Models and Techniques. Vol. 2.
        London: Pergamon Press.
Engel, F. L.
1980   Information selection from visual display units. Pp. 121-125
        in E. Grandjean and E. Vigliani, eds., Ergonomic Aspects of
        Visual Display Terminals. London: Taylor & Francis.
Erickson, R. A., Linton, P. M., and Hemingway, J. C.
1968   Human Factors Experiments with Television. Technical
        Report NWC TP 4573. China Lake, Calif.: Naval Weapons
        Center.
Ericsson, K. A., and Simon, H. A.
1980   Verbal reports as data. Psychological Review 87:215-251.
Evinger, D., Kaneko, C. R. S., Johanson, G. W., and Fuchs, A. F.
1977   Omnipauser cells in the cat. Pp. 337-340 in P. Baker and A.
        Berthoz, eds., Control of Gaze by Brainstem Neurons.
        Amsterdam: Elsevier.
Favilla, M., Ghelarducci, B., LaNoce, A., and Starita, A.
1981   Phase changes induced by ketamine in the verticle vestibulo
        ocular reflex in the rabbit. Brain Research 224:213-217.
Feldon, S. E., Stark, L., Lehman, S. L., and Hoyt, W. F.
1982   Oculomotor effects of intermittent conduction block in
        myasthenia gravis and Guillain-Barre syndrome: an
        oculographic study with computer simulations. Archives of
        Neurology 39:497-503.
Fellman, T. H., Brauninger, U., Gierer, R., and Grandjean, E.
1981   An Ergonomic Evaluation of VDTs. Report No. CH-8092.
        Zurich: Department of Hygiene and Ergonomics, Swiss
        Federal Institute of Technology.

Fender, D. H., and Nye, P. W.
   1961   An investigation of the mechanisms of eye movement
             control. Kybernetik 1:81-88.
Ferguson, D. A., Major, G., and Keldonlis, T.
   1974   Vision at work. Visual defect and the visual demand of
             tasks. Applied Ergonomics 5:84-93.
Ferri, E. S., and Hagan, G. J.
   1976   Chronic low-level exposure of rabbits to microwaves. Pp.
             129-142 in C. Johnson and M. Shore, eds., Biological Effects
             of Electromagnetic Waves. Vol. 1. (Selected papers of the
             USNC/URSI Annual Meeting, Boulder, Colorado, 1975.) HEW
             Publication (FDA)77-8010. Washington, D.C.: U.S.
             Department of Health, Education, and Welfare.
Fincham, E. F.
   1937   The mechanism of accommodation. British Journal of
             Ophthalmology Supplement 8:5-80.
   1951   The accommodation reflex and its stimulus. British Journal
             of Ophthalmology 35:381-393.
Fisher, D. F.
   1975   Reading and visual search. Memory and Cognition 3:188-196.
Frankenhaeuser, M.
   1980   Psychoendocrine approaches to the study of stressful person-
             environment transactions. Pp. 46-70 in H. Selye, ed., Selye's
             Guide to Stress Research. Vol. 1. New York: Van Nostrand.
Frankenhaeuser, M., and Gardell, B.
   1976   Underload and overload in working life: outline of a
             multidisciplinary approach. Journal of Human Stress
             2:35-46.
Frankenhaeuser, M., Nordheden, B., Myrsten, A. L., and Post, B.
   1971   Psychophysiological reactions to understimulation and
             overstimulation. Acta Psychologica 35:298-308.
French, J. R. P., Jr., and Caplan, R. D.
   1972   Organizational stress and individual strain. Pp. 30-66 in A.
             Morrow, ed., The Failure of Success. New York: AMOCOM.
French, J. R. P., Jr., and Kahn, R. L.
   1962   A programmatic approach to studying the industrial
             environment and mental health. Journal of Social Issues
             18:1-47.
French, J. R. P., Jr., Rodgers, W., and Cobb, S.
   1974   Adjustment as person-environment fit. Pp. 316-333 in G. V.
             Coelho, D. A. Hamburg, and J. E. Adams, eds., Coping and
             Adaptation. New York: Basic Books.
French, J. R. P., Jr., Caplan, R. D., and Harrison, R. V.
   1982   Mechanisms of Job Stress and Strain. New York: John Wiley
             & Sons.
Friedman, M., and Rosenman, R. H.
   1959   Association of specific covert patterns with blood and
             cardiovascular findings. Journal of the American Medical
             Association 169:1286-1296.
Friedman, M., Rosenman, R. H., and Carroll, V.
   1958   Changes in the serum cholesterol and blood clotting time in

men subjected to cyclic variation of occupational stress.
Circulation 18:852-861.

Fry, G. A., and King, V. M.
1975   The pupillary response and discomfort glare. Journal of the
Illuminating Engineering Society 4(4):307-324.

Frydman, M. I.
1981   Social support, life events and psychiatric symptoms: a
study of direct, conditional and interaction effects. Social
Psychiatry 16:69-78.

Fuchs, A. F. and Luschei, E. S.
1970   Firing patterns of abducens neurons of alert monkeys in
relationship to horizontal eye movements. Journal of
Neurophysiology 33:382-392.

Fugate, J. M., and Fry, G. A.
1956   Relation of changes in pupil size to visual discomfort.
Journal of the Illuminating Engineering Society 51:537-549.

Gardell, B.
1971   Alienation and mental health in the modern industrial
environment. Pp. 146-156 in L. Levi, ed., Society, Stress,
and Disease, I: The Psychosocial Environment and
Psychosomatic Diseases. London: Oxford University Press.

Gardner, G. T.
1978   Effects of federal human subjects regulations on data
obtained in environmental stressor research. Journal of
Personality and Social Psychology 36:628-634.

Gaskill, J. D.
1978   Linear Systems, Fourier Transforms and Optics. New York:
John Wiley & Sons.

Geacintov, T., and Peavler, W.
1974   Pupillography in industrial fatigue assessment. Journal of
Applied Psychology 59:213-216.

Ghiringelli, L.
1980   Collection of subjective opinions on use of VDU's. Pp.
227-231 in E. Grandjean and E. Vigliani, eds., Ergonomic
Aspects of Visual Display Terminals. London: Taylor &
Francis.

Ghiselli, E. E., and Brown, C. W.
1948   Personnel and Industrial Psychology. New York:
McGraw-Hill.

Glass, D.
1977   Behavior Patterns, Stress, and Coronary Disease. Hillsdale,
N. J.: Lawrence Erlbaum Associates.

Glass, D. C., and Singer, J. E.
1972   Urban Stress: Experiments in Noise and Social Stressors.
New York: Academic Press.

Gore, S.
1978   The effect of social support in moderating the health
consequences of unemployment. Journal of Health and
Social Behavior 19:157-165.

Gorrell, E. L.
1980   A Human Engineering Specification for Legibility of
Alphanumeric Symbology on Video Displays (Revised).
Technical Report No. 80-R-R-26. Downsview, Ontario:

Canadian Defence and Civil Institute of Environmental
Medicine (DCIEM).
Gosling, R. H.
1958   Peptic ulcer and mental disorder. Journal of Psychosomatic
         Research 2:284-301.
Granda, R. E.
1980   Man/machine design guidelines for the use of screen display
         terminals. Proceedings of the Human Factors Society 24th
         Annual Meeting 24:90-92.
Grandjean, E.
1980   Fitting the Task to the Man. London: Taylor & Francis.
1981   Sitzen Sie Richtig? Munich: Staatsministerium für Arbeit
         und Sozialordnung.
Grandjean, E. and Hunting, W.
1977   Ergonomics of posture. Review of various problems of
         standing and sitting posture. Applied Ergonomics 8:135-140.
Grandjean, E., and Vigliani, E., eds.
1980   Ergonomic Aspects of Visual Display Terminals. London:
         Taylor & Francis.
Grandjean, E., Nakoseko, M., Hunting, W., and Laubli, T.
1981   Ergonomic evaluation of a new type of keyboard. Zeitschrift
         fuer Arbeitswissenschaft 4:221-226. (In German)
Graybiel, A. M.
1977   Organization of oculomotor pathways in the cat and rhesus
         monkey. Pp. 79-88 in P. Baker and A. Berthoz, eds., Control
         of Gaze by Brainstem Neurons. Amsterdam: Elsevier.
Grieco, A., Moleni, G., Piccoli, B., and Perris, R.
1980   Field study in newspaper printing: a systematic approach to
         the VDU operator strain. Pp. 185-194 in E. Grandjean and E.
         Vigliani, eds., Ergonomic Aspects of Visual Display
         Terminals. London: Taylor & Francis.
Grieco, A., Occhipinti, E., Boccardi, S., Moleni, G., Colombini, D., and
Menoni, O.
1978   Development of a new method for evaluation of risks of
         injury induced by working posture. La Medicina del Lavoro
         (Supplement 3) 69:1-41.
Gunnarsson, E., and Soderberg, I.
1979   Work with Visual Display Terminals in Newspaper Offices.
         Report No. 1979-21. Stockholm: National Board of
         Occupational Safety and Health. (In Swedish.)
1980   Eyestrain Resulting from VDT Work at the Swedish
         Telecommunications Administration. Eye Changes and
         Visual Strain During Various Working Procedures.
         Stockholm: National Board of Occupational Safety and
         Health.
Guth, S. K.
1951   Brightness relationships for comfortable seeing. Journal of
         the Optical Society of America 41:235-244.
Guy, A. W., and Chou, C.-K.
1982   Hazard Analysis: Very Low Frequency Through Medium
         Frequency Range. Bioelectromagnetic Research Laboratory,
         Department of Rehabilitation Medicine. Seattle: University
         of Washington.

Haider, M., Kundi, M., and Weissenbock, M.
1980   Worker strain related to VDUs with differently coloured
        characters. Pp. 53-64 in E. Grandjean and E. Vigliani, eds.,
        Ergonomic Aspects of Visual Display Terminals. London:
        Taylor & Francis.
Halstead, W. C.
1941   A note on the Bartley effect in the estimation of equivalent
        brightness. Journal of Experimental Psychology 28:524-528.
Hammond, K. R., and Adelman, L.
1976   Science, values and human judgment. Science 194:389-396.
Harrison, R. V.
1976   Job Demands and Worker Health: Person-Environment
        Misfit. PhD dissertation. Department of Psychology,
        University of Michigan. (Dissertation Abstracts
        International 37:1035B)
1978   Person-environment fit and job stress. Pp. 175-205 in C. L.
        Cooper, and R. Payne, eds., Stress at Work. New York:
        John Wiley & Sons.
Heaton, J. M.
1966   The pain in eyestrain. American Journal of Ophthalmology
        61:104-112.
Hecht, S.
1934   Vision II. The nature of the photoreceptor process. Pp.
        704-828 in C. Murchison, ed., A Handbook of General
        Experimental Psychology. Worcester, Mass.: Clark
        University Press.
Helander, M. G.
1981   Review of Human Factors/Ergonomics Standards for Video
        Display Terminals. Paper presented at the Symposium on
        Video Display Terminals and Vision of Workers, Committee
        on Vision, National Research Council, Washington, D.C.,
        August.
Helander, M. G., Billingsley, P. A., and Schurick, J. M.
1983   An evaluation of human factors research on video display
        terminals in the work place. Human Factors Review 1.
Helmholtz, H.
1867   Handbuch der Physiologische Optik. Leipzig: Voss.
Henn, V., Cohen, B., and Young, L.
1980   Visual-Vestibular Interaction in Motion Perception and the
        Generation of Nystagmus. Cambridge, Mass.: MIT Press.
Hill, A. B.
1971   Principles of Medical Statistics. New York: Oxford
        University Press.
Hochberg, J.
1970   Components of literacy. Pp. 74-89 in H. Levin and J. P.
        Williams, eds., Basic Studies in Reading. New York: Basic
        Books.
Hoffman, A. C.
1946   Eye-movements during prolonged reading. Journal of
        Experimental Psychology 36:95-118.
Hofstetter, H. W.
1943   An ergographic analysis of fatigue and accommodation.
        American Journal of Optometry 20:115-135.

256

Holladay, L.
1926   The fundamentals of glare and visibility. Journal of the
        Optical Society of America 41:235-244.
Holland, M. K., and Tarlow, G.
1972   Blinking and mental load. Psychological Reports 31:119-127.
Hopkinson, R. G., and Collins, J. B.
1970   The Ergonomics of Lighting. London: MacDonald Technical
        and Scientific Press.
Horwitz, C., and Bronte-Stewart, B.
1962   Mental stress and serum lipid variation in ischemic heart
        disease. American Journal of Medical Science 244:272-281.
House, R. J., and Mitchell, T. R.
1975   Path-goal theory of leadership. Pp. 177-186 in K. N. Wexley
        and G. A. Yukl, eds., Organizational Behavior and Industrial
        Psychology. New York: Oxford University Press.
House, J. S.
1981   Work Stress and Social Support. Reading, Mass.:
        Addison-Wesley.
House, J. S., and Wells, J. A.
1978   Occupational stress, social support, and health. Pp. 8-29 in
        A. McLean, G. Black, and M. Colligan, eds., Reducing
        Occupational Stress: Proceedings of a Conference. HEW
        Publication No. (NIOSH) 78-140. Washington, D.C.: U. S.
        Department of Health, Education, and Welfare.
House, J. S., McMichael, A. J., Wells, J. A., Kaplan, B. H., and
Landerman, L. R.
1979   Occupational stress and health among factory workers.
        Journal of Health and Social Behavior 20:139-160.
Howe, L.
1916   The fatigue of accommodation, as registered by the
        ergograph. Journal of the American Medical Association
        67:100-104.
Huey, E. B.
1968   The Psychology and Pedagogy of Reading. Cambridge,
        Mass.: MIT Press. (Originally published 1908.)
Hultgren, G. V., and Knave, B.
1974   Discomfort glare and disturbances from light reflections in
        an office landscape with CRT display terminals. Applied
        Ergonomics 5(1):2-8.
Humes, J. M., and Bauerschmidt, D. K.
1968   Low Light Level TV Viewfinder Simulation Program. Phase
        B: The Effects of Television System Characteristics Upon
        Operator Target Recognition Performance. U.S. Air Force
        Avionics Laboratory Technical Report No. AFAL-TR-68-271.
        Dayton, Ohio: Wright-Patterson Air Force Base.
Hung, G., Hsu, F., and Stark, L.
1977   Dynamics of the human eyeblink. American Journal of
        Optometry. 54:678-690.
Hunting, W., Laubli, T., and Grandjean, E.
1981   Postural and visual loads at VDT workplaces. Ergonomics
        24:917-931.

Ilgen, D. R., and Seeley, W.
1974 Realistic expectations as an aid in reducing voluntary resignations. Journal of Applied Psychology 59:452-455.

International Business Machines
1979 Human Factors of Workstations with Display Terminals. 2d Ed. Document No. G320-6102-1. San Jose, Calif.: International Business Machines.

International Radiation Protection Association
1977 Overviews on Nonionizing Radiation. Rockville, Md.: Bureau of Radiological Health, U. S. Department of Health, Education, and Welfare.

Janis, I. L., and Mann, L.
1977 Decision Making: A Psychological Analysis of Conflict, Choice, and Commitment. New York: The Free Press.

Johansson, G., and Aronsson, G.
1980 Stress Reactions in Computerized Administrative Work. Reports from the Department of Psychology, University of Stockholm, Supplement Series. Supplement 50. Stockholm: University of Stockholm.

Johansson, G., Aronsson, G., and Lindstrom B. O.
1978 Social psychological and neuroendocrine stress reactions in highly mechanized work. Ergonomics 21:583-599.

Joreskog, K. G. and Sorbom, D.
1979 Advances in Factor Analysis and Structural Equation Models. Cambridge, Mass.: Abt Books.

Judd, C. H., and Buswell, G. T.
1922 Silent reading: a study of the various types. Supplementary Educational Monographs 23.

Just, M. A., and Carpenter, P. A.
1978 Inference processes during reading: reflections from eye fixations. Pp. 157-174 in J. W. Senders, D. F. Fisher, and R. A. Monty, eds., Eye Movements and the Higher Psychological Functions. Hillsdale, N.J.: Lawrence Erlbaum Associates.

Kahn, H. A., Leibowitz, H. M., Ganley, J. P.
1977 The Framingham eye study. 1. Outline and major prevalence findings. American Journal of Epidemiology 106:17.

Kahn, R. L.
1981 Work and Health. New York: John Wiley & Sons.

Kahn, R. L., and Quinn, R. P.
1970 Role stress: a framework for analysis. Pp. 50-115 in A. McLean, ed., Mental Health and Work Organizations. Chicago: Rand McNally.

Kahn, R. L., Wolfe, D. M. Quinn, R. P., Snoek, J. D. and Rosenthal, R. A.
1964 Organizational Stress: Studies in Role Conflict and Ambiguity. New York: John Wiley & Sons.

Kajiya, J., and Ullner, M.
1981 Filtering high quality text for display on raster scan devices. Computer Graphics 15:7-15.

Kasl, S. V.
1978 Epidemiological contributions to the study of work stress. Pp. 3-48 in C. L. Cooper and R. Payne, eds., Stress at Work. New York: John Wiley & Sons.

Katz, D., and Kahn, R. L.
1978   The Social Psychology of Organizations. New York: John
        Wiley & Sons.
Katzell, R. A., and Yankelovich, D.
1975   Work, Productivity, and Job Satisfaction. New York:
        Psychological Corporation.
Kaufman, J. E., and Christensen, J. F., eds.
1972   IES Lighting Handbook. 5th Ed. New York: Illuminating
        Engineering Society of America.
Keegan, J. J.
1953   Alternation of the lumbar curve related to posture and
        seating. Journal of Bone Joint Surgery 35:589-603.
Keller, E. L.
1977   Control of saccadic eye movements by midline brainstem
        neurons. Pp. 327-336 in P. Baker and A. Berthoz, eds.,
        Control of Gaze by Brainstem Neurons. Amsterdam:
        Elsevier.
Keller, E. L., and Robinson, D. A.
1972   Abducer unit behavior in the monkey during vergence
        movements. Vision Research 12:369-382.
Kenny, D. A.
1979   Correlation and Causality. New York: John Wiley & Sons.
King, V. M.
1972   Discomfort glare from flashing sources. Journal of the
        American Optical Association 43:53-56.
Kintz, R. T., and Bowker, D. O.
1982   Accommodation response during a prolonged visual search
        task. Applied Ergonomics 13:55-59.
Klein, M. V.
1970   Optics. New York: John Wiley & Sons.
Kohn, M. L., and Schooler, C.
1969   Class, occupation, and orientation. American Sociological
        Review 34:659-678.
Kolers, P. A., Duchnicky, R. L., and Ferguson, D. C.
1981   Eye movement measurement of readability of CRT displays.
        Human Factors 23:517-527.
Kramer, J.
1973   Biomechanische Veranderungen im Lumbalen
        Bewegungssegment. Stuttgart: Hippokrates Verlag.
Kraut, A. I.
1965   A Study of Role Conflicts and Their Relationships to Job
        Satisfaction, Tension, and Performance. Ph.D. dissertation.
        Department of Psychology, University of Michigan.
        (University Microfilms No. 66-06637)
Kravklov, S. V.
1974   The hygienic basis of standard of illumination. Types of
        visual fatigue. NASA Technical Translations 16(066):1-15.
Krishnan, V. V., Shirachi, D., and Stark, L.
1977   Dynamic measures of vergence accommodation. American
        Journal of Optometry and Physiological Optics 54:470-473.
Krishnan, V., and Stark, L.
1975   Integral control in accommodation. Computer Programs in
        Biomedicine 4:237-245.

Krivohlavy, J., Kodat, V., and Cizek, P.
1969   Visual efficiency and fatigue during the afternoon shift. Ergonomics 12:735-740.

Kroemer, K. H. E.
1970   Industrial Seating. Technical Paper AD 70-138. Detroit: Society of Mechanical Engineers.
1971   Seating in plant and office. American Industrial Hygiene Association Journal 32(10):633-642.
1972   Human engineering the keyboard. Human Factors 14:51-63.
1981   Engineering anthropometry: designing the work place to fit the human. Pp. 116-126 in Proceedings of the American Institute of Industrial Engineers Annual Conference. Norcross, Ga.: American Institute of Industrial Engineers.
1983   Engineering anthropometry: designing the work place to fit the user. In D. J. Oborne and M. M. Gruneberg, eds., Psychology and Productivity at Work: The Physical Environment. Chichester, England: John Wiley & Sons.

Kroemer, K. H. E. and Price, D. L.
1982   Ergonomics in the office: comfortable work stations allow maximum productivity. Industrial Engineering 14(7):24-32.

Krueger, H.
1980   Ophthalmological aspects of work with display workstations. Pp. 31-40 in E. Grandjean and E. Vigliani, eds., Ergonomic Aspects of Visual Display Terminals. London: Taylor & Francis.

Kulka, R. A.
1979   Interaction as person-environment fit. New Directions for Methodology of Behavioral Science 2:55-71.

Kurtz, J. I.
1937   The general and ocular fatigue problem. Parts I and II. American Journal of Optometry 14:273-308.
1938   An experimental study of ocular fatigue. I. General fatigue. American Journal of Optometry 15:86-117.

Lancaster, W. B., and Williams, E. R.
1914   New light on the theory of accommodation with practical applications. Transactions of the American Academy of Ophthalmology and Otolaryngology 19:170-195.

LaRocco, J. M., House, J. S., and French, J. R. P., Jr.
1980   Social support, occupational stress, and health. Journal of Health and Social Behavior 21:202-218.

Laubli, T., Hunting, W., and Grandjean, E.
1980   Visual impairments in VDU operators related to environmental conditions. Pp. 85-94 in E. Grandjean and E. Vigliani, eds., Ergonomic Aspects of Visual Display Terminals. London: Taylor & Francis.

Lazarus, R. S.
1966   Psychological Stress and the Coping Process. New York: McGraw-Hill.

Lee, R. E., and Schneider, R. F.
1958   Hypertension and arteriosclerosis in executive and nonexecutive personnel. Journal of the American Medical Association 167:1447-1450.

Leibowitz, H. W.
1977   Visual perception and stress. Pp. 25-37 in C. Borg, ed.,
        Physical Work and Effort. New York: Pergamon Press.
Leibowitz, H. W., and Owens, D. A.
1978   New evidence for the intermediate position of relaxed
        accommodation. Documenta Ophthalmologica 46(1);133-147.
Leo, J.
1980   Coping with computers. Discovery (December):95-97.
Levi, L.
1972   Stress and distress in response to psychosocial stimuli:
        laboratory and real life studies on sympathoadrenomedullary
        and related reactions. Acta Medica Scandinavica 191
        (Supplement 528):1-166.
Lilienfeld, A. M.
1971   Foundations of Epidemiology. New York: Oxford University
        Press.
Lion, K. S., and Brockhurst, R. J.
1951   Study of ocular movements under stress. Archives of
        Ophthalmology 46:315-318.
Liu, J., Lee, M., Jang, K., Ciuffreda, K., Wong, J., Grisham, D., and
Stark, L.
1979   Objective assessment of accommodation orthoptics. I.
        Dynamic insufficiency. American Journal of Optometry and
        Physiological Optics 56:285-294.
Lowenstein, O., Feinberg, R., and Loewenfeld, I. E.
1963   Pupillary movements during acute and chronic fatigue.
        Investigative Ophthalmology and Visual Science 2:138-157.
Lowenstein, O., and Loewenfeld, I. E.
1952   Disintegration of central autonomic regulation during
        fatigue and its reintegration by psychosensory controlling
        mechanisms. The Journal of Nervous and Mental Disease
        115(1):1-21.
Luckiesh, M.
1946   Comments on criteria of ease of reading. Journal of
        Experimental Psychology 36:180-182.
1947   Reading and the rate of blinking. Journal of Experimental
        Psychology 37:266-268.
Luckiesh, M., and Moss, F. K.
1935a   Muscular tension resulting from glare. Journal of General
        Psychology 8:455-460.
1935b   Fatigue of the extrinsic ocular muscles while reading under
        sodium and tungsten light. Journal of the Optical Society of
        America 25:216-217.
1937   The eyelid reflex as a criterion for ocular fatigue. Journal
        of Experimental Psychology 20:589-596.
1942   Reading as a Visual Task. New York: Van Nostrand.
Lulla, A. B., and Bennett, C. A.
1981   Discomfort glare: range effects. Journal of the Illuminating
        Engineering Society 10(2):74-80.
Lundberg, V., and Frankenhaeuser, M.
1978   Psychophysiological reactions to noise as modified by
        personal control over noise density. Biological Psychiatry
        6:51-59.

Lundervold, A. J. S.
   1951   Electromyographic investigations of position and manner of
           working in typewriting. Acta Physiologica Scandinavica
           24(Supplement 84): 1-171.
MacLeod, D. I. A.
   1978   Visual sensitivity. Annual Review of Psychology 29:613-646.
Maddock, R. J., Mollodot, M., Leat, S., and Johnson, C. A.
   1981   Accommodative responses and refractive error.
           Investigative Ophthalmology and Visual Science 20:387-391.
Mahto, R. S.
   1972   Eyestrain from convergence insufficiency. British Medical
           Journal 2:564-565.
Malmstrom, F. V., Randle, R. J., Murphy, M. R., Reed, L. E., and Weber,
R. J.
   1981   Visual fatigue: the need for an integrated model. Bulletin
           of the Psychonomic Society 17:183-186.
Mandal, A. C.
   1981   The seated man (Homo sedans). Applied Ergonomics
           12:19-26.
Matula, R. A.
   1981   Effects of VDU's on the eyes: a bibliography (1972-1980).
           Human Factors 23:581-586.
Mayer, A., and Barlier, A.
   1981   Conditions de Travail Devant les Ecrans Cathodiques. Etude
           de l'Environnement Lumineux. Report No. 1332-104-81.
           Paris: Institut National de Recherche et de Securite.
McConkie, G. W. and Rayner, K.
   1975   The span of the effective stimulus during a fixation in
           reading. Perception and Psychophysics 17:578-586.
   1976   Identifying the span of the effective stimulus in reading:
           literature review and theories of reading. Pp. 137-162 in H.
           Singer and R. B. Ruddell, eds., Theoretical Models and
           Processes of Reading. 2d Ed. Newark, Del.: International
           Reading Association.
McConville, J. T., Robinette, K. M., and Churchill, T.
   1981   An Anthropometric Data Base for Commercial Design
           Applications. Yellow Springs, Ohio: Anthropology Research
           Project.
McDowell, E. D., and Rockwell, T. H.
   1978   An exploratory investigation of the stochastic nature of the
           driver's eye movements and their relationship to the
           roadway geometry. Pp. 329-345 in J. W. Senders, D. F.
           Fisher, and R. A. Monty, eds., Eye Movements and the
           Higher Psychological Functions. Hillsdale, N.J.: Lawrence
           Erlbaum Associates.
McFarland, R. A., Holway, A. H., and Hurvich, L. M.
   1942   Studies of Visual Fatigue. Boston: Harvard Graduate School
           of Business Administration.
McGrath, J. E.
   1976   Stress and behavior in organizations. Pp. 1351-1396 in M.
           D. Dunnette, ed., Handbook of Industrial and Organizational
           Psychology. Chicago: Rand McNally.

McLeod, W. P., Mandel, D. R., and Malven, F.
  1980   The effects of seating on human tasks and perceptions. Pp.
           117-126 in Human Factors and Industrial Design in Consumer
           Products. Medford, Mass.: Tufts University.
Medalie, J. H., Snyder, M., Groen, J. J., Neufeld, H. N., Goldbourt, U.,
and Riss, E.
  1973   Angina pectoris among 10,000 men: 5-year incidence and
           univariate analysis. American Journal of Medicine.
           55:583-594.
Mershon, D. H., and Amerson, T. L., Jr.
  1980   Stability of measures of the dark focus of accommodation.
           Investigative Ophthalmology and Visual Science 19:217-221.
Microwave News
  1981   Birth defects and miscarriage clusters stir up more fears
           over VDTs. Microwave News 1(10):1-3.
Miles, R. H.
  1976   Role requirements as sources of organizational stress.
           Journal of Applied Psychology 61:172-179.
Miller, R. J.
  1978   Mood changes and dark focus of accommodation. Perceptual
           Psychophysics 24:437-443.
Milne, J. S., and Williamson, J.
  1972   Visual acuity in older people. Gerontologia Clinica
           14:249-256.
Moss, C. E., Murray, W. E., Parr, W. H., Messite, J., and Karches, G. J.
  1977   A Report on Electromagnetic Radiation Surveys of Video
           Display Terminals. Report No. DHEW (NIOSH) 78-129.
           Cincinnati: National Institute for Occupational Safety and
           Health.
Mourant, R. R., Lakshmanan, R., and Chantadisal, R.
  1981   Visual fatigue and cathode ray tube display terminals.
           Human Factors 23(5):529-540.
Murch, G.
  1982a   How visible is your display? Electro-Optical Systems
           Design. March:43-49.
  1982b   Visual fatigue with prolonged display use. Society for
           Information Display Digest 13:200-201.
Murray, H. A.
  1938   Explorations in Personality. New York: Oxford University
           Press.
Nachemson, A., and Elfstrom, G.
  1970   Intravital dynamic pressure measurements in lumbar discs.
           Scandinavian Journal of Rehabilitation Medicine (Supplement
           I).
National Council on Radiation Protection
  1977   Review of NCRP Radiation Dose Limit for Embryo and
           Fetus in Occupationally Exposed Women. NCRP Report No.
           53. Washington, D.C.: National Council on Radiation
           Protection.
National Council on Radiation Protection and Measures
  1981   Radiofrequency Electromagnetic Fields, Properties,
           Quantities, and Units, Biophysical Interaction and
           Measurements. NCRP Report No. 67. Washington, D. C.:
           National Council on Radiation Protection and Measures.

National Institute for Occupational Safety and Health
   1981   Potential Health Hazards of Video Display Terminals. DHHS
            (NIOSH) Publication No. 81-129. Cincinnati: National
            Institute for Occupational Safety and Health.
National Research Council
   1939   Conference on Visual Fatigue, May 20-21. Washington,
            D.C.: National Research Council.
   1980   The Effects on Populations of Exposure to Low Levels of
            Ionizing Radiation. Committee on the Biological Effects of
            Ionizing Radiation, Division of Medical Sciences, Assembly
            of Life Sciences. Washington, D. C.: National Academy
            Press.
   1981   Effects of Microwave Radiation on the Lens of the Eye.
            Working Group 35, Committee on Vision, Assembly of
            Behavioral and Social Sciences. Washington, D. C.: National
            Academy Press.
New York Committee for Occupational Safety and Health
   1980   Health Protection for Operators of VDTs/CRTs New York:
            New York Committee for Occupational Safety and Health.
Nilsen, A.
   1982   Facial rash in visual display unit operators. Contact
            Dermatitis 8(1):25-28.
Nisbett, R. E., and Wilson, T. D.
   1977   Telling more than we can know: verbal reports on mental
            processes. Psychological Review 84:231-259.
Noton, D., and Stark, L.
   1971a   Scanpaths in eye movements during pattern perception.
            Science 171:308-311.
   1971b   Eye movements and visual perception. Scientific American
            224:34-43.
   1971c   Scanpaths in saccadic eye movements while viewing and
            recognizing patterns. Vision Research 11:929-942.
Nowakowski, B.
   1926   The measurement of glare. American Journal of Hygiene
            6:1-31.
Nunnally, J. C.
   1967   Psychometric Theory. New York: McGraw-Hill.
O'Donnell, R. D., Gomer, F. E., Spicuzza, R. J., Renfroe, C. R., Klug, J.
A., and Bach, D. L.
   1976   Comparison of Human Information Processing Performance
            with Dot and Stroke Alphabetic Characters. Aerospace
            Medical Research Laboratory Report No. AMRL-TR-75-95.
            Dayton, Ohio: Wright-Patterson Air Force Base.
Olsen, R. A., ed.
   1981   Handbook for Design and Use of Visual Display Terminals.
            Sunnyvale, Calif.: Lockheed Missiles and Space Company.
Olsen, W. C.
   1981   Electric Field Enhanced Aerosol Exposure in Visual Display
            Unit Environments. Norwegian Directorate of Labor
            Inspection Report CMI No. 80364-1. Fantoft, Bergen,
            Norway: The Christian Michaelson Institute.
O'Neill, W. D. and Stark, L.
   1968   Triple function ocular monitor. Journal of the Optical
            Society of America 58:570-573.

Onishi, N., Nomura, H., and Sakai, L.
1973   Fatigue and strength of upper limb muscles of flight
        reservation system operators. Journal of Human Ergology
        2:133-141.

O'Regan, K.
1979   Moment to moment control of eye saccades as a function of
        textual parameters in reading. Pp. 49-60 in P. A. Kolers, M.
        E. Wrolstead, and H. Bouma, eds., Processing of Visible
        Language. New York: Plenum Press.

Östberg, O.
1978   Towards standards and threshold limit values for visual
        work. Pp. 359-382 in B. Tengroth and D. Epstein, eds.,
        Current Concepts of Ergophthalmology. Stockholm:
        International Ergophthalmological Society.
1980   Accommodation and visual fatigue in display work. Pp.
        41-52 in E. Grandjean and E. Vigliani, eds., Ergonomic
        Aspects of Visual Display Terminals. London: Taylor &
        Francis.

Östberg, O., Powell, J., and Blomkvist, A. C.
1980   Laser Optometry in Assessment of Visual Fatigue.
        University of Lulea Technical Report No. 1980:1T. Lulea,
        Sweden: University of Lulea.

Ostrom, C. A.
1981   Bussforares Arbetsmiljo: Stol. Report No. 229. Linkoping,
        Sweden: National Road and Traffic Institute.

Padmos, P., and Vos, J. J.
1980   The Validity of Interior Light Level Recommendations:
        Some Neglected Aspects. Publication No. 50. Paris:
        Commission Internationale de l'Eclairage.

Parrish, J. A., Anderson, R. A., Urbach, F., and Pitts, D. G.
1978   UV-A, Biological Effects of Ultraviolet Radiation with
        Emphasis on Human Response to Longwave Ultraviolet. New
        York: Plenum Press.

Paterson, D. G., and Tinker, M. A.
1956   Readability of newspaper headlines printed in capitals and
        lower case. Journal of Applied Psychology 30:161-168.

Pavlides, G. Th.
1981   Sequencing eye movements and the early objective diagnosis
        of dyslexia. Pp. 99-163 in G. Th. Pavlides and T. R. Miles,
        eds., Dyslexia Research and its Applications to Education.
        Chichester, England: John Wiley & Sons.

Pell, S., and D'Alonzo, C. A.
1963   A three-year study of myocardial infarction in a large
        employed population. Journal of the American Medical
        Association 175:463-470.

Peter, L. J., and Hull, R.
1969   The Peter Principle. New York: Morrow.

Petherbridge, P., and Hopkinson, R. G.
1955   A preliminary study of reflected glare. Transactions of the
        Illuminating Engineering Society 20:255-257.

Pflanz, M., Rosenstein, E., and Von Uexkull, T.
1956   Sociopsychological aspects of peptic ulcer. Journal of
        Psychosomatic Research 1:68-74.

Phillips, S., and Stark, L.
1977   Blur: a sufficient accommodative stimulus. Documenta
            Ophthalmologica 3:65-89.
Pinneau, S. R., Jr.
1975   Effects of Social Support on Psychological and Physiological
            Strain. PhD dissertation. Department of Psychology,
            University of Michigan.
Radl, G. W.
1980   Experimental investigations for optimal presentation-mode
            and colours of symbols on the CRT screen. Pp. 127-135 in E.
            Grandjean and E. Vigliani, eds., Ergonomic Aspects of Visual
            Display Terminals. London: Taylor & Francis.
Rashbass, C.
1959   Barbiturates, nystagmus and the mechanisms of visual
            fixation. Nature 183:897-898.
Rashbass, C., and Russel, G. F. M.
1961   Action of a barbiturate (amylobarbitone sodium) on the
            vestibulo ocular reflex. Brain 84:785-792.
Rayner, K.
1978   Eye movements in reading and information processing.
            Psychological Bulletin 85:618-660.
Reading, V. M., ed.
1978   Visual Aspects and Ergonomics of Visual Display Units.
            Department of Visual Science, Institute of Ophthalmology.
            London: University of London.
Reitmaier, J.
1979   Some effects of veiling reflections in papers. Lighting
            Research and Technology 11(4):204-209.
Rey, P., and Meyer, J. J.
1977   Problemes Visuels aux Ecrans de Visuelisation. Geneva,
            Switzerland: Groupe de Recherche sur les Ecrans de
            Visuelisation.
1980   Visual impairments and their objective correlates. Pp. 77-83
            in E. Grandjean and E. Vigliani, eds., Ergonomic Aspects of
            Visual Display Terminals. London: Taylor & Francis.
Ridder, C. A.
1959   Basic Design Measurement for Sitting. Agricultural
            Experiment Station Bulletin 116. Fayetteville: University
            of Arkansas.
Rinalducci, E. J.
1967   Early dark adaptation as a function of wavelength and
            pre-adapting level. Journal of the Optical Society of
            America 57:1270-1271.
Rinalducci, E. J., and Beare, A. N.
1974   Losses in nighttime visibility caused by transient
            adaptation. Journal of the Illuminating Engineering Society
            3:336-345.
1975   Visibility losses caused by transient adaptation at low
            luminance levels. Pp. 11-22 in Driver Visual Needs in Night
            Driving. Special Report 156. Transportation Research
            Board, Commission on Sociotechnical Systems, National
            Research Council. Washington, D.C.: National Academy of
            Sciences.

Riley, J. M., and Barbato, G. J.
1978   Dot-matrix alphanumerics viewed under discrete element degradation. Human Factors 20:473-479.

Roberts, J.
1978   Refraction Status and Motility Defects of Persons 4-74 Years, United States, 1971-1972. DHEW Publication No. (PHS) 78-1654. Washington, D. C.: U. S. Department of Health, Education, and Welfare.

Robinson, D. A.
1964   The mechanisms of human saccadic eye movements. Journal of Physiology 174:245-264.
1981   The use of control systems analysis in the neurophysiology of eye movements. Annual Review of Neuroscience 4:463-501.

Roebuck, J. A., Kroemer, K. H. E., and Thomason, W. G.
1975   Engineering Anthropometry Methods. New York: John Wiley & Sons.

Rohen, J. W., and Rentsch, F. J.
1969   Dur konstructiv bav des zonulaappartes beim manschen bund desser funktionelle bedertung. von Graefe's Archives of Clinical and Experimental Ophthalmology 178:1-19.

Rosenberg, M.
1968   The Logic of Survey Analysis. New York: Basic Books.

Roufs, J. A. J., and Bouma, H.
1980   Towards linking perception research and image quality. Proceedings of the Society for Information Display 21(3):247-270.

Rupp, B. A.
1981   Visual display standards: a review of issues. Proceedings of the Society for Information Display 22(1):63-72.

Russek, H. I.
1965   Stress, tobacco, and coronary heart disease in North American professional groups. Journal of the American Medical Association 192:189-194.

Saito, M., Tanaka, T., and Oshima, M.
1981   Eyestrain in inspection and clerical workers. Ergonomics 3:161-173.

Sakrison, D. J.
1977   On the role of the observer and a distortion measure in image transmission. IEEE Transactions on Communication COM-25:1251-1267.

Saladin, J. J., and Stark, L.
1975   Presbyopia: new evidence from impedance cyclography supporting the Hess-Goldstrand theory. Vision Research 15:537-541.

Sales, S. M.
1969   Organizational role as a risk factor in coronary disease. Administrative Science Quarterly 14:325-336.

Sauter, S. L., Arndt, R., and Gottlieb, M.
1981   A Controlled Survey of Working Conditions and Health Problems of VDT Operators at the New York Times. Unpublished report prepared for The Newspaper Guild. Department of Preventive Medicine, University of Wisconsin.

Schade, O. H.
1948   Electro-Optical Characteristics of Television Systems. RCA
        Review Vol. 11. Harrison, N.J.: Tube Department, RCA
        Victor.
Schaefer, D. J., Warren, W. B., and Cain, F. L.
1982   VLF Hazards Analysis. Final Technical Report Project
        A-3172, Biomedical Research Division, Electronics and
        Computer Systems Laboratory. Atlanta: Georgia Institute
        of Technology.
Schobert, H.
1962   Sitzhaltung, Sitzschaden, Sitzmobel. Berlin: Springer.
Scinto, L. F.
1978   Relation of eye fixation to old-new information of texts.
        Pp. 175-194 in J. W. Senders, D. F. Fisher, and R. A. Monty,
        eds., Eye Movements and the Higher Psychological
        Functions. Hillsdale, N.J.: Lawrence Erlbaum Associates.
Sekey, A. and Tietz, J.
1982   Text display by "saccadic scrolling." Visible Language
        16(1):62-77.
Shirachi, D., Liu, J., Lee, M., Jang, J., Wong, J., and Stark, L.
1978   Accommodation dynamics: 1. range nonlinearity. American
        Journal of Physiology 55:631-641.
Shurtleff, D. A.
1982   How to make displays legible. Contemporary Psychology
        27(1):46.
Sliney, D. H., and Wolbarsht, M. L.
1980   Safety with Lasers and Other Optical Sources, A
        Comprehensive Handbook. New York: Plenum Press.
Smith, A. B., Tanaka, S., and Halperin, W.
1982   A Preliminary Report on a Cross-Sectional Survey of VDT
        Users at the Baltimore Sun. Cincinnati: National Institute
        for Occupational Safety and Health.
Smith, F.
1971   Understanding Reading. New York: Holt, Rinehart and
        Winston.
Smith, M. J., Cohen, B. G. F., Stammerjohn, L. W., Jr., and Happ, A.
1981   An investigation of health complaints and job stress in video
        display operation. Human Factors 23:387-400.
Smith, M. J., Stammerjohn, L. W., Cohen, B. G. F., and Lalich, N. R.
1980   Job stress in video display operations. Pp. 201-209 in E.
        Grandjean and E. Vigliani, eds., Ergonomic Aspects of Visual
        Display Terminals. London: Taylor & Francis.
Smith, S. W., and Brown, D. G.
1971   Radiofrequency and Microwave Radiation Levels Resulting
        from Man-made Sources in the Washington, D. C. Area.
        Bureau of Radiological Health. DHEW Publication No.
        (FDA) 72-8015 BRHDEP 72-5. Washington, D. C.: U. S.
        Department of Health, Education, and Welfare.
Smith, W. J.
1966   Modern Optical Engineering. New York: McGraw-Hill.
1979   A review of literature relating to visual fatigue.
        Proceedings of the Human Factors Society 23rd Annual
        Meeting 23:362-366.

Snyder, H. L.
1974   Image quality and face recognition on a television display. Human Factors 16(3)300-307.

Snyder, H. L., and Maddox, M. E.
1978   Information Transfer from Computer-Generated Dot-Matrix Displays. Department of Industrial Engineering and Operations Research, Human Factors Laboratory Report No. HFL-78-3/ARO-78-1. Blacksburg, Va.: Virginia Polytechnic Institute and State University.

Snyder, H. L., and Taylor, G. B.
1979   The sensitivity of response measures of alphanumeric legibility to variations in dot matrix display parameters. Human Factors 21(4):457-471.

Sommer, A.
1977   Cataracts as an epidemiologic problem. American Journal of Ophthalmology 83:334-339.

1980   Epidemiology and Statistics for the Ophthalmologist. New York: Oxford University Press.

1981   Diabetes and senile cataract (letter). American Journal of Ophthalmology 92:134.

Sorsby, A.
1972   Modern Ophthalmology. Vol. 3. London: Butterworths Scientific Publications.

Spiro, R. J., Bruce, B. C., and Brewer, W. F., eds.
1980   Theoretical Issues in Reading Comprehension: Perspectives from Cognitive Psychology, Linguistics, Artificial Intelligence, and Education. Hillsdale, N.J.: Lawrence Erlbaum Associates.

Staffel, F.
1889   As quoted in Lundervold, A. J. S. 1951. Electromyographic investigations of position and manner of working in typewriting. Acta Physiologica Scandinavica 24(Supplement 84): 1-17.

Stammerjohn, L. W., Smith, M. J., and Cohen, B. G. F.
1981   Evaluation of work station design factors in VDT operations. In M. J. Smith, B. G. F. Cohen, L. W. Stammerjohn, and A. Happ, eds., An Investigation of Health Complaints and Job Stress in Video Display Operations. Cincinnati: National Institute for Occupational Safety and Health.

Stark, L.
1968   Neurological Control Systems. New York: Plenum Press.

1971   The control system for versional eye movements. Pp. 363-428 in P. Bach-y-Rita, C. C. Collins, and J. E. Hyde, eds., The Control of Eye Movements. New York: Academic Press.

1975   The main sequence, a tool for studying human eye movements. Mathematical Biosciences 24:191-204.

Stark, L., and Bahill, A. T.
1979   The trajectories of saccadic eye movements. Scientific American 240:108-117.

Stark, L., and Ellis, S. R.
1981   Scanpaths revisited: cognitive models direct active

looking. Pp. 193-116 in D. F. Fisher, R. A. Monty, and J. W. Senders, eds., Eye Movements, Cognition and Visual Perception. Hillsdale, N. J.: Lawrence Erlbaum Associates.

Stark, L., Vossius, G., and Young, L.
1962 Predictive control of eye tracking movements. Institute of Radiation Engineering. IRE Transactions, Human Factors in Electronics HFE 3:52-57.

Stark, L., Hoyt, W., Ciuffreda, K., Kenyon, R. and Hsu, F.
1980 Time optimal saccadic trajectory model and voluntary nystagmus. Pp. 75-89 in B. L. Zuber, ed., Models of Ocular Motor Behavior and Control. Boca Raton, Fla: CRC Press.

Stein, I. H.
1980 The effect of active area on the legibility of dot-matrix displays. Proceedings of the Society for Information Display 21:17-20.

Stern, J.
1978 Eye movements, reading, and cognition. Pp. 145-155 in J. W. Senders, D. F. Fisher, and R. A. Monty, eds., Eye Movements and the Higher Psychological Functions. Hillsdale, N.J.: Lawrence Erlbaum Associates.

Stewart, T. F. M.
1980a Practical experiences in solving VDU ergonomic problems. Pp. 233-240 in E. Grandjean and E. Vigliani, eds., Ergonomic Aspects of Visual Display Terminals. London: Taylor & Francis.
1980b Problems caused by continuous use of visual display units. Lighting Research and Technology 12:26-36.

Stodgill, R. M.
1974 Handbook of Leadership. New York: Free Press.

Swedish National Board of Occupational Safety and Health
1979 Reading of Display Screens. Health Directive 136. Stockholm: Swedish National Board of Occupational Safety and Health.

Tannenbaum, A. S., Kavcic, B., Rosner, M., Vianello, M., and Wieser, R.
1974 Hierarchy in Organizations. San Francisco: Jossey-Bass.

Task, H. L., and Verona, R. W.
1976 A New Measure of Television Display Quality Relatable to Observer Performance. Aerospace Medical Research Laboratory Report No. AFAMRL-TR-76-73. Dayton, Ohio: Wright-Patterson Air Force Base.

Taylor, H. R.
1980 The environment and the lens. British Journal of Ophthalmology 64:303.
1981 Racial variations in vision. American Journal of Epidemiology 113:62-80.
1982 The author replies. American Journal of Epidemiology 115:139-142.

Teele, R. P.
1965 Photometry. Pp. 1-42 in R. Kingslake, ed., Applied Optics and Optical Engineering. Vol. 1. New York: Academic Press.

ten Doesschate, J. and Alpern, M.
1967 The effect of photoexcitation of the two retinas on pupil size. Journal of Neurophysiology 30:562-576.

Terrana, T., Merluzzi, F., and Giudici, E.
1980   Electromagnetic radiations emitted by visual display units.
         Pp. 13-21 in E. Grandjean and E. Vigliani, eds., Ergonomic
         Aspects of Visual Display Terminals. London: Taylor &
         Francis.
Terreberry, S.
1968   The evolution of organizational environments.
         Administrative Science Quarterly 12:590-614.
Tichauer, E. R.
1976   Biomechanics sustains occupational safety and health.
         Industrial Engineering 27:46-56.
Timmers, H., van Nes, F. L., and Blommaert, F. J. J.
1980   Visual word recognition as a function of contrast. Pp.
         115-120 in E. Grandjean and E. Vigliani, eds., Ergonomic
         Aspects of Visual Display Terminals. London: Taylor &
         Francis.
Tinker, M. A.
1939   The effect of illumination intensities upon speed of
         perception and upon fatigue in reading. Journal of
         Educational Psychology 30:561-571.
1946   Validity of frequency of blinking as a criterion of
         readability. Journal of Experimental Psychology 36:453-460.
1949   Involuntary blink rate and illumination intensity in visual
         work. Journal of Experimental Psychology 39:558-560.
1965   Legibility of Print. Ames: Iowa State University Press.
Tinker, M. A., and Paterson, D.
1939   Influence of type form on eye movements. Journal of
         Experimental Psychology 25:528-531.
Toffler, A.
1970   Future Shock. New York: Random House.
Tomizuka, M., and Whitney, D. E.
1975   Optimal finite pre-preview problems (why and how is future
         information important?). ASME Journal of Dynamic
         Systems, Measurement and Control 97(4):319-325.
Treurniet, W. C.
1980   Spacing of characters on a television display. Pp. 365-374 in
         P. A. Kolers, M. E. Wrolstead, and H. Bouma, eds.,
         Processing of Visible Language. New York: Plenum Press.
Troelstra, A.
1968   Detection of time-varying light signals as measured by the
         pupillary response. Journal of the Optical Society of
         America 58:685-690.
Troup, J. D. G.
1978   Postural stress in sedentary work. Pp. 51-62 in V. M.
         Reading, ed., Visual Aspects and Ergonomics of Visual
         Display Units. London: Institute of Ophthalmology,
         University of London.
United Nations Scientific Committee on the Effects of Atomic Radiation
1977   Sources and Effects of Ionizing Radiation. USCEAR Report
         to the General Assembly, with annexes. New York: United
         Nations.

U.S. Army Environmental Hygiene Agency
    1981   Investigation of Adverse Pregnancy Outcomes Defense
             Contract Administration Services Region, Atlanta, GA.
             Occupational Health Special Study No. 66-32-1359-81.
             Alexandria, Va.: Defense Logistics Agency.

U.S. Department of Defense
    1971   Human Factors Engineering Design for Army Materiel.
             MIL-HDBK-759. Washington, D.C.: U.S. Department of
             Defense.
    1974   Human Engineering Design Criteria for Military Systems,
             Equipment and Facilities. MIL-STD-1472B. Washington,
             D.C.: U.S. Department of Defense.
    1981   Human Engineering Design Criteria for Military Systems,
             Equipment and Facilities. MIL STD 1472C. Washington,
             D.C.: U.S. Department of Defense.

Usui, S., and Stark, L.
    1978   Sensory and motor mechanisms interact to control amplitude
             of pupil noise. Vision Research 18:505-507.

Van Cott, H. P., and Kinkade, A. G., eds.
    1972   Human Engineering Guide to Equipment Design. Catalog No.
             D210.6/2:En2. Washington, D.C.: U.S. Government Printing
             Office.

van Heyningen, R.
    1975   What happens to the human lens in cataract. Scientific
             American 233:70-81.

van Nes, F. L., and Bouman, M. A.
    1967   Spatial modulation transfer in the human eye. Journal of the
             Optical Society of America 57:401-406.

van Wely, P.
    1970   Design and disease. Applied Ergonomics 1:262-264.

Vernon, H.
    1924   As quoted in Lundervold, A. J. S. 1951. Electromyographic
             investigations of position and manner of working in
             typewriting. Acta Physiologica Scandinavica 24(Supplement
             84):1-17.

Vroom, V. H., and Yetton, P. W.
    1973   Leadership and Decision-Making. Pittsburgh: University of
             Pittsburgh Press.

Walker, C. R., and Guest, R. H.
    1952   The Man on the Assembly Line. Cambridge, Mass.: Harvard
             University Press.

Wanous, J. P.
    1978   Realistic job previews: can a procedure to reduce turnover
             also influence the relationship between abilities and
             performance? Personnel Psychology 31:249-258.

Warwick, D. P., and Lininger, C. A.
    1975   The Sample Survey: Theory and Practice. New York:
             McGraw-Hill.

Watanabe, A., Mori, T., Nagata, S., and Hiwatashi, K.
    1968   Spatial sine-wave responses of the human visual system.
             Vision Research 8:1245-1263.

Weber, R. A.
    1950   Ocular fatigue. Archives of Ophthalmology 43:257-264.

Weiss, M. W., and Petersen, R. C.
1979   Electromagnetic radiation emitted from video computer
        terminals. American Industrial Hygiene Association Journal
        40(4):300-309.
Westheimer, G.
1957   Accommodation measurements in empty visual fields.
        Journal of the Optical Society of America 47:714-718.
1963   Amphetamines, barbiturates, and accommodation-vergence.
        AMA Archives of Ophthalmology 70:830-836.
Westheimer, G., and Rashbass, C.
1961   Barbiturates and eye vergence. Nature 191:833-834.
Whiteside, T. C. D.
1957   The Problems of Vision in Flight at High Altitude. London:
        Butterworths Scientific Publications.
Wilkinson, I. M. S., Kime, R., and Purnell, M.
1974   Alcohol and human eye movement. Brain 97:785-792.
Williams, T. P., and Baker, B. N., eds.
1980   The Effects of Constant Light on the Visual Process. New
        York: Plenum Press.
Wilson, V., and Jones, G. M.
1979   Mammalian Vestibular Physiology. New York: Plenum
        Press.
Wolbarsht, M. L., O'Foghludha, F. A., Sliney, D. H., Guy, A. W., Smith, A.
A., Jr., and Johnson, G. A.
1980   Electromagnetic emission from visual display units: a
        non-hazard. Pp. 187-195 in M. L. Wolbarsht and D. H.
        Sliney, eds., Ocular Effects of Non-Ionizing Radiation.
        (Proceedings of the Society of Photo-Optical
        Instrumentation Engineers, Vol. 229.) Bellingham, Wash.:
        Society of Photo-Optical Instrumentation Engineers.
Wood, C. L., and Bitterman, M. E.
1950   Blinking as a measure of effort in visual work. American
        Journal of Psychology 63:584-588.
Woodson W. E.
1981   Human Factors Design Handbook. New York: McGraw-Hill.
Woodworth, R. S.
1938   Experimental Psychology. New York: Holt, Rinehart and
        Winston.
Working Women Education Fund
1981   Warning: Health Hazards for Office Workers. Cleveland, Ohio:
        Working Women Education Fund.
Working Women, National Association of Office Workers
1980   Race Against Time: Automation of the Office. Cleveland:
        Working Women, National Association of Office Workers.
World Health Organization
1979   Ultraviolet Radiation. Environmental Health Criteria
        Document No. 14. Geneva: World Health Organization.
1981   Microwave Radiation. Environmental Health Criteria
        Document No. 17. Geneva: World Health Organization.
Yamaguchi, Y., Umezawa, F., and Jashinada, Y.
1972   Sitting posture: an electromyographic study on health and
        notalgic people. Journal of Japanese Orthopedic Association
        46:51-56.

Yarbus, A. L.
1967   Eye Movements and Vision. New York: Plenum Press.
Yonemura, G. T.
1977   Task lighting--another view. Lighting Design and
        Application (November):27-30.
Young, L., and Stark, L.
1963   Variable feedback experiment testing a sampled data model
        for eye tracking movements. IEEE Transactions on Human
        Factors in Electronics HFE 4:38-51.
Zaret, M. M.
1980a   Cataracts and visual display units. Pp. 49-60 in Proceedings
        of the Conference on Health Hazards of VDUs.
        Loughborough, England: Loughborough University of
        Technology.
1980b   Cataracts Following Use of Cathode Ray Tube Displays.
        Paper presented at the International Symposium of
        Electromagnetic Waves and Biology, Juoy-en-Josas, France,
        June 30-July 4, 1980.
1981   Testimony presented before the Subcommittee on
        Investigations and Oversight, Committee on Science and
        Technology, U. S. House of Representatives, Washington,
        D.C., May 12, 1981.
Zentralstelle für Unfallverhutung und Arbeitsmedizin
1980   Hauptuerband der gewerblichen Berufsgenossenschaffen e. V.
        (Safety Regulations for Display Workplaces in the Office
        Sector.) Köln, W. Germany: Carl Heymanns Verlag KG.
Zigman, S., and Vaughan, T.
1974   Near ultraviolet light effects on the lenses and retinas of
        mice. Investigative Ophthalmology and Visual Science
        13:462-465.
Zigman, S., Datiles, M., and Torcyznski, E.
1979   Sunlight and human cataracts. Investigative Ophthalmology
        and Visual Science 18:462-467.
Zipp, P., Ohl, B., Haider, E., and Rohmert, W.
1980   EMG Untersuchungen der Korperhaltung bei der Variation
        von Tastaturparametern. Pp. 257-259 in W. Brenner, J.
        Rutenfranz, E. Baumgartner, and M. Haider, eds.,
        Arbeitsbedingte: Gesundheitsschaden-Fiktion Oder
        Wirklichkeit. Stuttgart: Genter.